Current Clinical Strategies

Anesthesiology

1999-2000 Edition

Mark R. Ezekiel, MD, MS

Current Clinical Strategies Publishing

www.ccspublishing.com

Digital Book and Updates

Purchasers of this book can download the digital book and updates at the Current Clinical Strategies Publishing internet site: www.ccspublishing.com

© 1999, 2000 Current Clinical Strategies Publishing. All rights reserved. This book, or any parts thereof, may not be reproduced, photocopied, or stored in an information retrieval network without the written permission of the publisher. The reader is advised to consult the drug package insert and other references before using any therapeutic agent. No warranty exists, expressed or implied, for errors or omissions in this text.

Current Clinical Strategies is a registered trademark of Current Clinical Strategies Publishing.

> Current Clinical Strategies Publishing Inc
> 27071 Cabot Road
> Laguna Hills, California 92653
> Phone: 800-331-8227
> Fax: 800-965-9420
> Internet: www.ccspublishing.com
> E-mail: info@ccspublishing.com

Printed in USA   ISBN 1-881528-71-5

Table of Contents

Cardiopulmonary Resuscitation and Advanced Cardiac Life Support	5
Preoperative Evaluation	11
Cardiovascular Disease	16
Pulmonary Disease	19
Endocrinology	20
Liver Disease	25
Chemotherapy	25
Basics of Anesthesiology	27
Medical Gas Systems	27
Electrical Safety	27
Anesthesia Machine	28
Patient Monitors	29
Anesthesia Machine Check	31
Pharmacology	34
Cardiovascular Physiology	72
Respiratory Physiology	83
Airway Management	87
Laboratory Values	96
Fluid and Electrolyte Management	97
Blood Therapy Management	98
Spinal and Epidural Anesthesia	104
Regional Anesthesia	107
Pediatric Anesthesia	110
Cardiac Surgery	114
Vascular Surgery	121
Thoracic Surgery	124
Obstetrical Anesthesia	127
Neuroanesthesia	133
Pain Management	138
Trauma	142
Ophthalmologic Surgery	146
Transurethral Resection of the Prostate	148
Electroconvulsive Therapy	148
Laparoscopic Surgery	149
Myasthenia Gravis	149
Myasthenic Syndrome	150
Anesthesia for Organ Harvest	150
Postanesthesia Care Unit	152
Malignant Hyperthermia	154
Allergic Drug Reactions	156
Venous Air Embolism	156
Latex Allergy	157
References	159
Index	160

Cardiopulmonary Resuscitation and Advanced Cardiac Life Support

Universal Algorithm for Adult Emergency Cardiac Care

1. Assess responsiveness.
2. Activate EMS (emergency medical services) system. Call for defibrillator.
3. Assess breathing (open the airway, look, listen, and feel). If the patient is not breathing, give two slow breaths.
4. Assess circulation
   A. If there is a pulse, categorize the patient to one of the following suspected causes, and then go to the appropriate algorithm.
      1. Hypotension; shock; acute pulmonary edema.
      2. Acute myocardial infarction.
      3. Arrhythmia that is either too fast or too slow.
   B. If there is no pulse
      1. Start CPR and check monitor for ventricular fibrillation (VF) or ventricular tachycardia (VT), if VF/VT go to algorithm.
      2. Otherwise, intubate, confirm tube placement and ventilations, and determine rhythm and cause.
      3. If there is electrical activity with no pulse, go to the pulseless electrical activity algorithm.

Ventricular Fibrillation/Pulseless Ventricular Tachycardia Algorithm

1. Airway, breathing, and circulation (ABCs). CPR until defibrillator available.
2. Defibrillate.
   A. 200 J (unsynchronized).
   B. 200-300 J (unsynchronized).
   C. 360 J (unsynchronized).
3. CPR, IV, intubate. Continue if persistent or recurrent VF/VT.
4. Epinephrine, 1:10,000, 1.0 mg IVP, repeat every 3-5 minutes.
   A. Alternative epinephrine dosing
      1. Intermediate dose: epinephrine 2-5 mg IVP every 3-5 min.
      2. Escalating dose: epinephrine 1 mg, 3 mg, and 5 mg IVP given 3 minutes apart.
      3. High dose: epinephrine 0.1 mg/kg IVP, repeat every 3-5 min.
5. Defibrillate 360 J (unsynchronized) within 30-60 seconds.
6. Lidocaine 1.5 mg/kg IVP, repeat every 3-5 minutes to a total loading dose of 3 mg/kg; then use:
   A. Bretylium, 5 mg/kg IV, repeat with 10 mg/kg every 15-30 minutes to total of 30 mg/kg.
   B. Magnesium sulfate 1-2 grams IV in Torsades de Pointes or suspected hypomagnesemic state or severe refractory VF.
   C. Procainamide 30 mg/min in refractory ventricular fibrillation (maximum total 17 mg/kg).

6 Cardiopulmonary Resuscitation

7. Defibrillate 360 J, 30-60 seconds after each dose of medications.
8. Consider bicarbonate 1 mEq/kg (if known preexisting bicarbonate responsive acidosis, overdose with tricyclic antidepressant).

Asystole Algorithm

1. Airway, breathing, and circulation (ABCs). CPR, intubate, start IV.
2. Confirm asystole in two or more leads. If rhythm is unclear and possible ventricular fibrillation, defibrillate as for VF.
3. Consider possible causes: hypoxia, hyperkalemia, hypokalemia, preexisting acidosis, drug overdose, and hypothermia.
4. Consider immediate transcutaneous pacing.
5. Epinephrine, 1:10,000, 1.0 mg IVP, repeat every 3-5 minutes.
    A. Alternative epinephrine dosing
        1. Intermediate dose: epinephrine 2-5 mg IVP every 3-5 min.
        2. Escalating dose: epinephrine 1 mg, 3 mg, and 5 mg IVP given 3 minutes apart.
        3. High dose: epinephrine 0.1 mg/kg IVP, repeat every 3-5 min.
6. Atropine 1.0 mg IV, repeat every 3-5 minutes to total of 0.04 mg/kg.
7. Consider bicarbonate 1 mEq/kg (if known preexisting bicarbonate responsive acidosis, overdose with tricyclic antidepressants, prolonged arrest, hypoxic lactic acidosis).

Pulseless Electrical Activity Algorithm

1. Pulseless electrical activity includes: idioventricular rhythms, ventricular escape rhythms, postdefibrillation idioventricular rhythms.
2. Airway, breathing, and circulation (ABCs).
3. Initiate CPR, intubate, start IV.
4. Consider possible causes: pericardial tamponade, tension pneumothorax, hypovolemia, massive pulmonary embolus, hypoxia, hypothermia, drug overdose (such as tricyclics, digitalis, beta blockers, calcium channel blockers), hyperkalemia, acidosis, massive acute myocardial infarction.
5. Epinephrine, 1:10,000, 1.0 mg IVP, repeat every 3-5 minutes.
    A. Alternative epinephrine dosing
        1. Intermediate dose: epinephrine 2-5 mg IVP every 3-5 min.
        2. Escalating dose: epinephrine 1 mg, 3 mg, and 5 mg IVP given 3 minutes apart.
        3. High dose: epinephrine 0.1 mg/kg IVP, repeat every 3-5 min.
6. If absolute bradycardia (<60 bpm) or relative bradycardia, give atropine 1 mg IVP every 3-5 minutes up to a total of 0.04 mg/kg.
7. Consider bicarbonate 1 mEq/kg (if known preexisting bicarbonate responsive acidosis, overdose with tricyclic antidepressants, prolonged arrest, hypoxic lactic acidosis).

Bradycardia Algorithm

1. Heart rate <60 beats/minute. Mechanisms include: sinus or junctional, second degree AV block type I or II, third degree AV block.
2. Airway, breathing, and circulation (ABCs).
3. Administer oxygen, start IV, place monitors.
4. If time allows review history, examine patient, 12 lead EKG, portable CXR.
5. If unstable (considered unstable if chest pain, shortness of breath, decreased level of consciousness, hypotension, shock, pulmonary congestion, congested heart failure or acute myocardial infarction are present).
   A. Atropine 0.5-1.0 mg IVP repeated every 3-5 minutes up to 0.04 mg/kg (denervated transplanted hearts will not respond to atropine, go immediately to transcutaneous cardiac pacing).
   B. Transvenous pacing: If patient is symptomatic, do not delay transcutaneous cardiac pacing while awaiting IV access or atropine effect.
   C. Dopamine 5-20 mcg/kg/min.
   D. Epinephrine 2-20 mcg/min.
   E. Isoproterenol 0.5-20 mcg/min.
6. If stable and not in type II or type III AV heart block, observe.
7. If type II or type III AV heart block, prepare for transvenous pacer (never treat third-degree heart block plus ventricular escape beats with lidocaine).

Tachycardia Algorithm

1. Support airway, breathing, and circulation (ABCs).
2. Administer oxygen; secure airway; start IV, assess vital signs.
3. If time allows review history, examine patient, 12 lead EKG, portable CXR.
4. If unstable (chest pain, hypotension, CHF, myocardial infarction, ischemia, decreased level of consciousness, shock, dyspnea or pulmonary congestion).
   A. If ventricular rate is greater than 150, consider immediate cardioversion.
   B. Consider brief trial of medications based on arrhythmia.
5. If stable treat according to arrhythmia.
   A. Atrial fibrillation/atrial flutter. Consider diltiazem, beta blockers, verapamil, procainamide, quinidine, anticoagulants.
   B. Paroxysmal supraventricular tachycardia (PSVT)
      1. Vagal maneuvers (carotid sinus pressure is contraindicated in patients with carotid bruits; avoid ice water immersion in patients with ischemic heart disease).
      2. Adenosine 6 mg rapid IVP (over 1-3 seconds); may repeat with 12 mg rapid IVP in 1-2 minutes for a total of 30 mg.
      3. Check QRS complex width
         A. If normal complex width
            1. Verapamil 2.5-5.0 mg slow IV, repeat with 5-10 mg in 15-30 minutes if no response.
            2. Consider beta blockers, diltiazem, digoxin.
            3. Consider synchronized cardioversion.

8 Cardiopulmonary Resuscitation

    B. If wide complex width
        1. Lidocaine 1-1.5 mg/kg IVP.
        2. Procainamide 20-30 mg/min, to total of 17 mg/kg.
        3. Consider synchronized cardioversion.
    C. Wide complex tachycardia of uncertain type
        1. Lidocaine 1-1.5 mg/kg IVP, repeat every 5-10 minutes with 0.5-0.75 mg/kg, up to maximum total of 3 mg/kg.
        2. Adenosine 6 mg rapid IVP; may repeat with 12 mg rapid IVP in 1-2 min for total of 30 mg.
        3. Procainamide 20-30 mg/min, to total of 17 mg/kg.
        4. Bretylium 5-10 mg/kg IV over 8-10 minutes, maximum total 30 mg/kg over 24 hours.
        5. Consider synchronized cardioversion.
    D. Stable ventricular tachycardia
        1. Lidocaine 1-1.5 mg/kg IVP, repeat every 5-10 minutes with 0.5-0.75 mg/kg, up to maximum total of 3 mg/kg.
        2. Procainamide 20-30 mg/min, to total of 17 mg/kg.
        3. Bretylium 5-10 mg/kg IV over 8-10 minutes, maximum total 30 mg/kg over 24 hours.
        4. Consider synchronized cardioversion.

Electrical Cardioversion Algorithm

1. Consider in tachycardia with serious signs and symptoms related to the tachycardia (seldom needed for ventricular rates less than 150 beats/min).
2. Check oxygen saturation, suction, IV line, airway equipment.
3. Premedicate whenever possible.
4. Synchronized cardioversion (note if conditions are critical, go immediately to unsynchronized cardioversion).
   A. For VT, atrial fib/flutter use 100 J, 200 J, 300 J, 360 J.
   B. For PSVT (and sometimes atrial flutter) start with 50 J.

Ventricular Ectopy

1. Assess need for acute suppression therapy: rule out treatable causes, consider serum potassium, digitalis levels, bradycardia or drug induced.
2. Lidocaine 1 mg/kg.
3. If not suppressed, repeat lidocaine 0.5 mg/kg every 2-5 minutes until no ectopy or up to total of 3 mg/kg.
4. If not suppressed, procainamide 20 mg/min until no ectopy or up to total of 1000 mg.
5. If not suppressed, bretylium 5-10 mg/kg over 8 minutes.
6. If not suppressed, consider overdrive pacing.

Maintenance Drips

1. After lidocaine dose of 1 mg/kg: start lidocaine drip at 2 mg/min.
2. After lidocaine dose of 1-2 mg/kg: start lidocaine drip at 3 mg/min.

Cardiopulmonary Resuscitation

3. After lidocaine dose of 2-3 mg/kg: start lidocaine drip at 4 mg/min.
4. After loading dose of procainamide: start procainamide drip at 1-4 mg/min.
5. After loading dose of bretylium: start bretylium drip at 2 mg/min.

Drugs That May Be Given Endotracheally

ALIEN V
1. Atropine, Lidocaine, Isoproterenol, Epinephrine, Naloxone, and Valium.

Newborn Resuscitation

1. The major cause of cardiac arrest is hypoxemia due to airway obstruction and respiratory depression.
2. Airway management
   A. Positive-pressure ventilation should be started for apnea, cyanosis, and heart rates below 100 beats/min.
   B. Assisted ventilation should be continued until spontaneous respirations are present and the heart rate is greater than 100 beats/min.
3. Chest compression
   A. The sternum is depressed 0.5-0.75 inch at a rate of 120 beats/min. The compression-ventilation ratio in neonates is 3:1.
   B. Heart rates below 60 beats/min chest compressions should be started.
   C. Heart rates 60-80 beats/min should be evaluated after ventilation with 100% oxygen has been performed for 30 seconds. If heart rate is not rising or is below 80 beats/min, chest compression should be started.

Pediatric ACLS Drugs		
Drug	Dose	Remarks
Adenosine	0.1-0.2 mg/kg	Give rapid IV bolus; max single dose 12 mg
Atropine	0.01-0.02 mg/kg Min dose: 0.1 mg	Max single dose: 0.5 mg in child, 1.0 mg in adolescent
Bretylium	5 mg/kg (may be increased to 10 mg/kg)	Give rapid IV Loading dose
Calcium Chloride 10%	20 mg/kg per dose	Give slowly
Dopamine	2-20 mcg/kg/min	Titrate to desired effect
Dobutamine	2-20 mcg/kg/min	Titrate to desired effect

10 Cardiopulmonary Resuscitation

Drug	Dose	Remarks
Epinephrine	First dose: IV/IO: 0.01 mg/kg (1:10k) ET: 0.1 mg/kg (1:1000); doses as high as 0.2 mg/kg may be effective Subsequent doses: IV/IO/ET: 0.1 mg/kg	Epinephrine infusion: 0.05-1.0 mcg/kg/min titrate to desired effect
Lidocaine	1 mg/kg per dose	Infuse 20-50 mcg/kg/min
Narcan	0.01 mg/kg	
Sodium Bicarbonate	1-2 mEq/kg per dose or 0.3 x kg x base deficit	Infuse slowly
Valium	0.1-0.25 mg/kg	
Defibrillation	2-4 watt-sec/kg	
Cardioversion	0.25-1.0 watt-sec/kg	

Preoperative Evaluation

I. The goal of the preoperative evaluation is to identify and correct conditions in order to reduce perioperative morbidity and mortality and alleviate patient anxiety.

II. **Anesthesia preoperative interview**
   A. Note the date and time of the interview, the planned procedure, and a description of any extraordinary circumstances regarding the anesthesia.
   B. **Current medications and allergies.** History of steroids or chemotherapy should be noted.
   C. Cigarette, alcohol, and drug history, including most recent use.
   D. **Anesthetic history**, including specific details of any problems.
   E. **Prior surgical procedures** and hospitalizations.
   F. **Family history**, especially anesthetic problems. Birth and development history (pediatric cases).
   G. **Obstetrical history:** last menstrual period (females).
   H. **Medical problems** previously diagnosed; evaluation, current treatment, and degree of control.
   I. **Review of systems,** including cardiac, pulmonary, or neurologic disease, reflux, or bleeding tendency.
   J. **Exercise tolerance.**
   K. History of airway problems (difficult intubation or airway disease, symptoms of temporomandibular joint disease, loose teeth).
   L. Physical exam, including airway evaluation, current vital signs, height and body weight, baseline mental status, evaluation of heart and lungs, vascular access.
   M. Overall impression of the complexity of the patient's medical condition, with assignment of ASA Physical Status Class.
   N. Anesthetic plan (general anesthesia, regional, spinal). The anesthetic plan is based on the patient's medical status, the planned operation, and the patient's wishes.
   O. Documentation that risks and benefits were explained to the patient.

III. **Preoperative laboratory evaluations**
   A. **Hemoglobin.** Menstruating females, children less than 1 year old or with suspected sickle cell disease, history of anemia, blood dyscrasia or malignancy, congenital heart disease, chronic disease states, age greater than 60 years, patients likely to experience significant blood loss.
   B. **WBC count.** Suspected infection or immunosuppression.
   C. **Platelet count.** History of abnormal bleeding or bruising, liver disease, blood dyscrasias, chemotherapy, hypersplenism.
   D. **Coagulation studies.** History of abnormal bleeding, anticoagulant drug therapy, liver disease, malabsorption, poor nutrition.
   E. **Electrolytes, blood glucose, BUN/creatinine.** Patients with hypertension, diabetes, heart disease, or disease states with potential for fluid-electrolyte abnormalities. Blood tests performed within 6 months of surgery that show normal results can be used if there has been no intervening clinical event, age greater than 60 years.
   F. **Liver function tests**. Patients with liver disease, history of or exposure to hepatitis, history of alcohol or drug abuse, drug therapy with agents that may affect liver function.
   G. **Pregnancy test.** Patients in whom pregnancy cannot be reliably ruled out by history.

12 Preoperative Evaluation

- **H. Electrocardiogram.** Men over age 40, women over age 55, history or symptoms of cardiac disease, history of diseases associated with cardiac involvement (hypertension, diabetes, morbid obesity, peripheral vascular disease, collagen vascular disease, cocaine abuse). An EKG showing normal results that was performed within 6 months of surgery can be used if there has been no intervening clinical event.
- **I. Chest x-ray.** Patients with symptoms of pulmonary disease, airway obstruction, cardiac disease, malignancy, history of heavy smoking, age greater than 60 years. A study showing normal results that was performed within one year of surgery can be used if there has been no intervening clinical event.
- **J. Urinalysis.** No indication in preanesthetic evaluation; surgeon may request to rule out infection before certain surgical procedures.
- **K. Cervical spine flexion/extension.** Patients with rheumatoid arthritis or Down's syndrome.
- **L. Preoperative pulmonary function tests (PFTs)**
    1. There is no evidence to suggest that pulmonary function tests are useful for purposes of risk assessment or modification in patients with cigarette smoking or adequately treated brochospastic disease.
    2. Candidates for preoperative PFTs
        a. Patients considered for pneumonectomy.
        b. Patients with moderate to severe pulmonary disease scheduled for major abdominal or thoracic surgery.
        c. Patients with dyspnea at rest.
        d. Patients with chest wall and spinal deformities.
        e. Morbidity obese patients.
        f. Patients with airway obstructive lesions.

IV. Airway evaluation

- **A. Medical conditions associated with difficult intubations**
    1. **Arthritis.** Patients with arthritis may have a decreased range of neck mobility. Rheumatoid arthritis patients have an increased risk of atlantoaxial subluxation.
    2. **Morbid obesity** patients have an increased incidence of sleep apnea.
    3. **Tumors** may obstruct the airway or cause extrinsic compression and tracheal deviation.
    4. **Infections** of any oral structure may obstruct the airway.
    5. **Trauma** patients are at increased risk for cervical spine injuries, basilar skull fractures, intracranial injuries, and facial bone fractures.
    6. **Down's Syndrome** patients may have atlantoaxial instability and macroglossia.
    7. **Scleroderma** may result in decreased range of motion of the temporomandibular joint and narrowing of the oral aperture.

V. Predictors of difficult intubation

- **A.** Obesity, buckteeth, large tongue, decreased jaw movement, receding mandible or anterior larynx, short stout neck.
- **B. Physical exam**
    1. **Anatomic variations.** Micrognathia, prognathism, large tongue, arched palate, short neck, prominent upper incisors.
    2. **Mouth**
        a. Oral opening size. Patients should be able to open their mouth at least 3 finger breadths.
        b. Poor dentition or loose teeth increase the risk of dental damage

and dislodgement.
   c. Macroglossia will increase difficulty of intubation.
3. Neck
   a. **Anterior mandibular space.** Estimated by measuring the distance between the hyoid bone and the inside of the mentum or between the notch of the thyroid cartilage to the mentum. An inadequate mandibular space is associated with a hyoid-mentum distance of less than 3 cm or a thyroid notch-mentum distance of less than 6 cm.
   b. **Cervical spine mobility (atlantooccipital joint extension).** Thirty-five degrees of extension are possible at the normal atlantooccipital joint
   c. Presence of a healed or patent tracheostomy stoma.
4. Airway classification
   a. Mallampati classification
      (1) **Class 1:** Able to visualize the soft palate, fauces, uvula, anterior and posterior tonsillar pillars.
      (2) **Class 2:** Able to visualize the soft palate, fauces, and uvula. The anterior and posterior tonsillar pillars are hidden by the tongue.
      (3) **Class 3:** Only the soft palate and base of uvula are visible.
      (4) **Class 4:** Only the soft palate can be seen (the uvula is not visualized).
   b. Grades of laryngoscopic view
      (1) **Grade 1:** Visualization of the entire laryngeal aperture.
      (2) **Grade 2:** Visualization of just the posterior portion of the laryngeal aperture.
      (3) **Grade 3:** Visualization of only the epiglottis.
      (4) **Grade 4:** Visualization of just the soft palate.

VI. **American Society of Anesthesiology (ASA) physical status classification**
   A. The ASA physical status has been shown to generally correlate with the perioperative mortality rate (mortality rates by ASA classification are given below).
   B. **ASA 1:** A normal healthy patient (0.06-0.08%).
   C. **ASA 2:** A patient with a mild systemic disease (mild diabetes, controlled hypertension, obesity) (0.27-0.4%).
   D. **ASA 3:** A patient with a severe systemic disease that limits activity (angina, COPD, prior myocardial infarction) (1.8-4.3%).
   E. **ASA 4:** A patient with an incapacitating disease that is a constant threat to life (CHF, renal failure) (7.8-23%).
   F. **ASA 5:** A moribund patient not expected to survive 24 hours (ruptured aneurysm) (9.4-51%).
   G. **ASA 6:** Brain-dead patient whose organs are being harvested.
   H. **For emergent operations,** add the letter E after the classification.

VII. **Preoperative fasting guidelines** (hours)

Age	Clear Liquids	Food/Milk
Prem/Newborn	2	4
1-6 months	2	4
7-36 months	3	6
3-15 years	3	8
Adults	8	8

14 Bacterial Endocarditis Prophylaxis

    A. Clear liquids include water, sugar-water, apple juice, non-carbonated soda (not pulp-containing juices, milk, etc).
    B. Medications can be taken with a small amount of a clear liquid).
VIII. Premedications
    A. Premedications are commonly given to alleviate patient anxiety.
    B. Healthy adults generally do not require premedications. Patients for cardiac surgery, however, typically receive premedications.
    C. Sedatives and analgesics should be reduced or withheld in the elderly, debilitated, and acutely intoxicated, as well as those with upper airway obstruction or trauma, central apnea, neurologic deterioration, or severe pulmonary or valvular heart disease.

Commonly Used Premedications

Classification	Drug	Adult (mg)	Peds (mg/kg)	Route
Barbiturates	Pentobarbital	50-150	2	IM
	Secobarbital		2	IM
	Methohexital		8	IM
	Methohexital		25-30	PR
Non-barbiturates	Ketamine		2-4	IM
	Ketamine		3	Intranasal
	Ketamine		6-10	PO
Opioids	Fentanyl		0.01-0.02	IM, IV
	EMLA		2.5 gm	Transdermal
	Sufentanil		0.0015-.0003	Intranasally
	Morphine	5-15	0.05-0.2	IM
	Meperidine	50-100	1-1.5	IM
Benzodiazepines	Diazepam	5-10	0.2-0.4	PO
	Midazolam	2.5-5		IM
	Midazolam		0.2-0.5	Intranasally
	Midazolam		0.4-1.0	PO
	Midazolam	0.2		SL
	Midazolam		0.5-1.0	PR
	Lorazepam	1-4		PO, IV
Non-benzo	Chloral Hydrate		30-50	PO/PR
Antihistamines	Benadryl	25-75		PO, IM
	Phenergan	25-50	0.5	IM
	Vistaril	50-100	0.5-1.0	IM
Anticholinergic	Atropine	0.3-0.6	0.02	IM, IV
	Scopolamine	0.3-0.6	0.008	IM, IV
	Glycopyrrolate	0.2-0.3	0.004-0.008	IM, IV
H_2 blockers	Cimetidine	200-400		PO, IM, IV
	Ranitidine	150-300		PO
	Ranitidine	50		IV
Antacids	Bicitra	15-60 cc		PO
Gastric stim	Metoclopramide	10-20		PO, IV, IM

Bacterial Endocarditis Prophylaxis

I. **Antibiotic prophylaxis** is recommended for patients with prosthetic cardiac valves, previous history of endocarditis, most congenital malformations, rheumatic valvular disease, hypertrophic cardiomyopathy, and mitral valve regurgitation.

II. Antibiotics for dental, oral or upper respiratory tract procedures

A. Oral regimen. Amoxicillin: 3 gm PO 1 hr before procedure, then 1.5 gm PO 6 hr after initial dose.

B. Oral regimen for penicillin-allergic patients
1. Erythromycin. 1 gm PO 2 hr before procedure, then 500 mg PO after initial dose.
2. Clindamycin. 300 mg PO 1 hr before procedure, then 150 mg PO 6 hr after dose.

C. IV regimen. Ampicillin. 2 gm IV 30 min before procedure, then 1 gm IV 6 hr after initial dose.

D. IV regimen for penicillin-allergic patients. Clindamycin. 300 mg PO 1 hr before procedure, then 150 mg PO 6 hr after dose.

E. High-risk patients. Ampicillin, gentamicin, and amoxicillin. ampicillin, 2 gm IV, plus gentamicin, 1.5 mg/kg, 30 min before procedure; followed by amoxicillin, 1.5 PO 6 hr after initial dose, or ampicillin, 2 gm IV, and gentamicin, 1.5 mg/kg 8 hr after initial dose.

F. High-risk penicillin-allergic patients
1. Vancomycin. 1 gm IV 1 hr before the procedure.

III. Antibiotics for genitourinary or gastrointestinal tract procedures

A. Standard regimen. Ampicillin, gentamicin, and amoxicillin: ampicillin, 2 gm IV, plus gentamicin, 1.5 mg/kg, 30 min before procedure; followed by amoxicillin, 1.5 PO 6 hr after initial dose.

B. Penicillin-allergic patients
1. Vancomycin and gentamicin. Vancomycin 1 gm IV, gentamicin 1.5 mg/kg IV, 1 hr before the procedure; repeat 8 hr after initial dose.

Cardiovascular Disease

I. **Preoperative risk factors.** The two most important predictors of cardiac morbidity are a history of recent (within 6 months) myocardial infarction and evidence of congestive heart failure.

II. **Primary cardiac risk factors**
  A. **Congestive heart failure.**
  B. **Angina.**
  C. **Previous myocardial infarction.** Increased reinfarction rates for 6 months after MI. Mortality after perioperative MI 20-50%. Infarction rate in the absence of a prior MI 0.13%.
  D. **Hypertension.** Risk factor for cardiac disease, but not independently associated with increased risk of perioperative MI.
  E. **Dysrhythmias.** Ventricular dysrhythmia may indicate underlying cardiac disease. Isolated premature ventricular contractions without evidence of underlying cardiac disease are not associated with increased cardiac risk.
  F. **Prior cardiac surgery.** a history of prior coronary artery bypass surgery or coronary angioplasty does not increase perioperative risk.

III. **Secondary risk factors** include diabetes mellitus, cigarette smoking, hypercholesterolemia, age, genetics, and vascular disease.

IV. **Contraindications to elective noncardiac surgery** include a myocardial infarction less than 1 month prior to surgery, uncompensated heart failure, and severe aortic or mitral stenosis.

V. **Ischemic heart disease**
  A. **Preoperative management**
    1. Patients with extensive three-vessel or left main disease, a history of myocardial infarction, or ventricular dysfunction are at risk for cardiac complications. Patients with history of myocardial infarction less than 6 months previously appear to be at greatest risk.
    2. **History**
        a. The most important symptoms to elicit include chest pain, dyspnea, poor exercise tolerance, syncope, or near-syncope.
        b. In patients with prior myocardial infarction or angina, localization of the areas of ischemia is invaluable in deciding which electrocardiographic leads to monitor intraoperatively.
    3. **Laboratory evaluation**
        a. Baseline EKG is normal in 25-50% of patients with coronary artery disease but no prior myocardial infarction. EKG evidence of ischemia often becomes apparent only during chest pain.
    4. **Noninvasive studies**
        a. **Exercise stress testing.** Gives estimate of functional capacity along with the ability to detect EKG changes and hemodynamic response. Highly predictive when ST-segment changes are characteristic of ischemia.
        b. **Echocardiography.** Evaluates global and regional ventricular function, valvular function, and congenital abnormalities. Detects regional wall motion abnormalities and derives left ventricular ejection fraction.
        c. **Dobutamine stress echo.** Reliable predictor of adverse cardiac complications.
        d. **Technetium-99m.** Extremely sensitive and specific for acute MI and for evaluating cardiac function.

Cardiovascular Disease

      e. Coronary angiography. Gold standard for evaluating cardiac disease. The single most important measurement is the ejection fraction.

B. Anesthetic considerations
1. **Premedications.** Premedications help reduce fear, anxiety and pain, and help prevent sympathetic activation.
2. **Cardiac medications.** Generally continued up until the time of surgery.
3. **Supplemental oxygen** should be given to all patients with significant ischemia or who are given sedation.
4. **Monitoring**
   a. **EKG.** Usually, lead II is monitored for inferior wall ischemia and arrhythmias and V_5 for anterior wall ischemia.
   b. The sudden appearance of a prominent v wave on the wedge waveform is usually indicative of acute mitral regurgitation from ischemic papillary muscle dysfunction or acute left ventricular dilation.
   c. **Maintenance anesthesia.** Patients with good ventricular function are generally managed with volatile agents, while those with depressed ventricular function are usually managed with an opioid based anesthetic.

VI. Hypertension
A. Preoperative evaluation
1. The perioperative history should assess the severity and duration of the hypertension, drug therapy, and the presence of hypertensive complications.
2. Surgical procedures on patients with sustained preoperative diastolic blood pressures higher than 110 mmHg or with evidence of end-organ damage should be delayed until blood pressure is controlled.
3. Premedications reduce preoperative anxiety. Cardiac and hypertensive medications should be continued up until the time of surgery.

B. Anesthetic considerations
1. Many patients with hypertension display an accentuated hypotensive response to induction followed by an exaggerated hypertensive response to intubation.
2. Techniques used to attenuate the hypertensive response include deepening anesthesia with a volatile agent, giving a bolus of narcotic, lidocaine or a beta blocker.

VII. Heart transplantation
A. Physiology of cardiac transplantation
1. The transplanted heart is totally denervated and direct autonomic influences are absent. Resting heart rate, in the absence of vagal influences, is increased (100-120 beats/min).
2. Cardiac output tends to be low normal and meets demand by increasing stroke volume and subsequently by increasing heart rate in response to circulating catecholamines.
3. Drugs that act via the autonomic system are ineffective.
4. Beta-adrenergic receptors remain intact.

B. Preoperative evaluation
1. Evaluation should focus on functional status (activity level) and detecting complications of immunosuppression.
2. Underlying cardiac disease may be asymptomatic because of the denervation.

18 Cardiovascular Disease

   3. Baseline EKG may demonstrate multiple P waves and a right bundle branch block.
C. **Anesthetic considerations**
   1. Maintain preload.
   2. Sudden vasodilation should be avoided because reflex increases in heart rate are absent. Indirect vasopressors are less effective than direct acting agents because of the absence of catecholamine stores in myocardial neurons
   3. Increases in heart rate are not seen following atropine.

Pulmonary Disease

I. Pulmonary risk factors
  A. **Risk factors** include preexisting pulmonary disease, thoracic or upper abdominal surgery, smoking, obesity, age greater than 60 years, and prolonged general anesthesia.
  B. The two strongest predictors of complications are operative site and a history of dyspnea.
  C. **Smoking**. Cessation of smoking for 24-48 hours before surgery may reduce carboxyhemoglobin levels. Cessation for greater than 4 weeks is required to reduce the risk of postoperative pulmonary complications.

II. Asthma
  A. **Preoperative**
   1. Asthma is characterized by airway hyperreactivity, manifest by episodic attacks of dyspnea, cough, and wheezing.
   2. Preoperative evaluation should ascertain the severity and control of the asthma, drug therapy, previous steroid use and history of intubation.
   3. Patients should be medically optimized prior to surgery. Patients with active bronchospasm presenting for emergency surgery should undergo a period of intensive treatment whenever possible.
   4. Bronchodilators should be continued up to the time of surgery. Theophylline levels should be checked preoperatively. Patients receiving steroids should be given supplemental doses (hydrocortisone 100 mg).

  B. **Intraoperative management**
   1. The most critical time is during instrumentation of the airway. Deep anesthesia should be accomplished prior to intubation and surgical stimulation of the airway.
   2. Reflex bronchospasm can be blunted prior to intubation by increasing the depth of anesthesia with additional induction agent or volatile agent, or by administering IV or intratracheal lidocaine.
   3. Intraoperative bronchospasm is usually manifest by wheezing, increasing peak airway pressure, decreased exhaled tidal volumes or a slowly rising wave form on the capnograph. Treatment should include deepening the level of anesthesia, and beta adrenergic agonists delivered by aerosol or metered dose inhalers.
   4. Patients should be extubated either before airway reflexes return or after the patient is fully awake. Lidocaine may help suppress airway reflexes during emergence.

III. Chronic obstructive pulmonary disease (COPD)
  A. Preoperative evaluation should involve the same approach as that used in the asthmatic.
  B. Routine pulmonary function tests are not recommended.
  C. A history of frequent exacerbations, steroid dependence, or need for intubation for respiratory support should prompt particular caution in the evaluation and planning for surgery.
  D. Choice of anesthetic technique should be geared toward minimizing complications. If general anesthesia is required, airway manipulation should be avoided to decrease bronchospasm.

Endocrinology

Diabetes Mellitus

I. **Regimens for perioperative glucose and insulin management**
   A. **Patients taking an oral agent**
      1. Sulfonylurea agents should be withheld within 24 hours of surgery. Other oral agents can be given until the patient is placed NPO.
      2. Glucose should be checked before and after the procedure.
   B. **Insulin-treated type 2 diabetics**
      1. Patients should receive half their normal morning insulin dose. A glucose-containing infusion should be started.
      2. Blood glucose should be checked before and after the procedure.
   C. **Insulin-treated type 1 diabetics**
      1. Patients must receive insulin to prevent ketoacidosis.
      2. Insulin can be given by sliding scale or continuous infusion.
         a. Regular insulin. 50 U/250 cc NS = 0.2 units/cc (flush IV tubing before starting).
         b. Insulin rate in U/hr = blood glucose/150 (use 100 as denominator if patient is on steroids, or is markedly obese, or infected). Alternative dosing. 0.1 units/kg/hr.

II. **Day of surgery.** Continue D5W and insulin infusion (for patients undergoing major surgery consider rechecking plasma glucose and potassium on morning of surgery).
   A. Check blood glucose at the start of surgery and every hour intraoperatively. Adjust insulin infusion as needed to keep glucose levels between 100-200 mg/dL.

III. **Other medications/Information**
   A. One can estimate the soluble (regular) insulin requirement by taking the daily dose of lente units and multiplying by 1.5. This gives the units of regular insulin required per day.
      1. One unit of insulin (IV) will lower the blood sugar by 30-40 mg/dL in a 70 kg person.
      2. Ten grams of dextrose will raise the blood sugar by 30-40 mg/dL in an average 70 kg person.
      3. Premeds. Zantac (50 mg IVPB) and metoclopramide (10 mg); (consider Bicitra 30 cc).
      4. One in four insulin dependent diabetics may have "stiff joint syndrome" and may be difficult to intubate.
      5. Diabetics may have gastroparesis as a result of autonomic neuropathy. The drug of choice for a nauseated or vomiting diabetic is metoclopramide 10 mg IV.
      6. In obstetrics, the insulin requirements may drop after delivery.
      7. Lactate is converted to glucose in the liver. Lactated Ringers may cause a blood glucose elevation.

Endocrinology 21

Types of Insulin			
Drug	Onset	Peak Action	Duration
Humalog	5-15 min	1 hour	3.5-4.5 hours
Regular	15-30 min	1-3 hours	5-7 hours
Semilente	30-60 min	4-6 hours	12-16 hours
Lente, NPH	2-4 hours	8-10 hours	18-24 hours
Ultralente	4-5 hours	8-14 hours	24-36 hours

Oral Hypoglycemic Agents		
Drug	Onset (hrs)	Duration (hrs)
Tolbutamide (Orinase)	0.5-1	6-12
Acetohexamide (Dymelor)	0.5-1	12-24
Tolazamide (Tolinase)	4-6	10-18
Chlorpropamide (Diabinese)	24-72	60-90
Glyburide (Micronase)	0.5-1	24-60
Glipizide (Glucotrol)	1-3	12-24

Pheochromocytoma

I. **Definition.** Catechol-secreting tumors usually located in an adrenal gland. Most pheochromocytomas produce both norepinephrine and epinephrine. Endogenous catecholamine levels should return to normal levels within 1-3 days after successful removal of the tumor. Overall mortality: 0-6%.

II. **Clinical manifestations**
   A. **Triad of symptoms.** Palpitations, headaches, and diaphoresis.
   B. **Signs.** Paroxysmal hypertension (hallmark).
   C. **Other manifestations** include flushing, anxiety, tremor, hyperglycemia, polycythemia, and weight loss.
   D. **Diagnosis** is confirmed by abnormally high levels of catecholamines or catechol metabolites in urine. Assay of 24 hour urinary metanephrine is the most reliable indicator of excess catecholamine secretion.

III. **Preoperative evaluations**
   A. **Prazosin or phenoxybenzamine** may be used to produce preoperative alpha-adrenergic blockade. Ten to 14 days are usually required for

adequate alpha-receptor blockade. Beta blockade is instituted after the onset of adequate alpha blockade if dysrhythmias or tachycardia persists.
  B. **Preoperative goals** include blood pressure below 160/95, no ST-T wave changes, and maximum of one PVC per 5 minutes.
IV. **Anesthetic considerations**
  A. **Overall goal** is to avoid sympathetic hyperactivity.
  B. **Drugs to avoid**
    1. Histamine releasers. Morphine, curare, atracurium.
    2. Vagolytics and sympathomimetics. Atropine, pancuronium, gallamine, succinylcholine.
    3. Myocardial sensitizers. Halothane.
    4. Indirect catechol stimulators. Droperidol, ephedrine, TCAs, chlorpromazine, glucagon, metoclopramide.
  C. **Monitors.** Intraarterial catheter in addition to standard monitors.
  D. **Combined technique** (general with spinal or epidural) is effective in ablating sympathetic responses while providing good muscle relaxation.
  E. **Preoperative normalization of fluid status** is essential in limiting hypotension following tumor resection.

Hyperthyroidism

I. **Clinical manifestations** may include: Weight loss, heat intolerance, muscle weakness, diarrhea, hyperactive reflexes, nervousness, exophthalmos, sinus tachycardia/atrial fibrillation and fine tremors.
II. **Management of anesthesia**
  A. **Preoperative.** All elective surgery should be postponed until the patient is rendered euthyroid with medical treatment. Preoperative assessment should include normal thyroid function tests, and a resting heart rate less than 85-90 beats/min. The combined use of beta antagonists and potassium iodide is effective in rendering most patients euthyroid in 10 days.
  B. **Intraoperative.** Thiopental is the induction agent of choice, since it possesses some antithyroid activity. Drugs that will stimulate the sympathetic nervous system should be avoided (ketamine, pancuronium, indirect-acting adrenergic agonists, etc.). MAC requirements for inhaled agents or anesthetic requirements are not increased with hyperthyroidism. Cardiovascular function and body temperature should be closely monitored.
  C. **Postoperative.** Most serious postoperative problem is thyroid storm, which is characterized by hyperpyrexia, tachycardia, altered consciousness, and hypotension. Most commonly occurs 6-24 hours postoperatively. Treatment includes hydration and cooling; propranolol (0.5 mg increments until heart rate is below 100 beats/min); propylthiouracil (250 mg every 6 hours orally) followed by sodium iodide (1 gm IV over 12 hours); and correction of any precipitating cause.
  D. **Complications after total or partial thyroidectomy.** Recurrent laryngeal nerve palsy, hematoma formation, hypothyroidism, and

hypoparathyroidism.

Hypothyroidism

I. **Clinical manifestations** may include generalized reduction in metabolic activity, lethargy, intolerance to cold, weight gain, constipation and decreased cardiac function.

II. **Myxedema coma** results from extreme hypothyroidism and is characterized by impaired mentation, hypoventilation, hypothermia, hyponatremia, and congested heart failure. Treatment is with IV thyroid hormones (300-500 mcg of levothyroxine sodium in patients without heart disease).

III. **Management of anesthesia**
   A. **Preoperative.** Patients with uncorrected severe hypothyroidism or myxedema coma should not undergo elective surgery. Mild to moderate hypothyroidism is not a absolute contraindication to surgery. Patients should be treated with histamine H_2 blockers and metoclopramide because of their slowed gastric emptying times.
   B. **Intraoperative.** Ketamine is the induction agent of choice because of the exquisite sensitivity of hypothyroid patients to drug-induced myocardial depression. MAC requirements for inhaled agents are not changed with hypothyroidism.
   C. **Postoperative.** Recovery from general anesthesia may be delayed by slowed drug biotransformation, hypothermia, and respiratory depression.

Obesity

I. **Definitions**
   A. Overweight is defined as up to 20% more than predicted ideal body weight.
   B. Obesity is defined as more than 20% above ideal body weight.
   C. Morbid obesity is defined as more than twice as much as their ideal body weight.

II. **Body mass index**
   A. Clinically the most useful index for defining obesity.
   B. Body mass index (BMI) = weight (kg)/height^2 (meters squared).
   C. A BMI greater then 28 kg/m^2 defines obesity; BMI greater than 35 kg/m^2 defines morbid obesity.

III. **Clinical manifestations**
   A. **Cardiovascular.** Systemic hypertension, cardiomegaly, congestive heart failure, coronary artery disease. Cardiac output increases by 0.1 L/min/kg of adipose tissue.
   B. **Ventilation.** Decreased lung volumes and capacities (suggestive of restrictive lung disease), arterial hypoxemia (decreased functional residual volume predisposes the obese patient to a rapid decrease in PaO$_2$), obesity-hypoventilation syndrome, decreased chest wall compliance.

C. Liver. Abnormal liver function tests, fatty liver infiltration.
D. Metabolic. Insulin resistance (diabetes mellitus), hypercholesterolemia.
E. Gastrointestinal. Hiatal hernia, gastroesophageal reflux.

IV. Obesity-hypoventilation syndrome (Pickwickian syndrome)
A. Occurs in 8% of obese patients, most commonly in the extremely obese.
B. Obstructive sleep apnea consists of episodes of nasal and oral airflow obstruction during sleep despite continuing respiratory effort. Obstruction is generally due to backward tongue movement and pharyngeal wall collapse (glossoptosis) secondary to interference with the normal coordinated contraction of pharyngeal and hypopharyngeal muscles.
C. Characterized by hypercapnia, cyanosis-induced polycythemia, right-sided heart failure, and somnolence. The presence of episodic daytime somnolence and hypoventilation in a morbidly obese patient suggests the presence of this syndrome.
D. Obstructive sleep apnea is diagnosed by finding at least 30 episodes of apnea (at least 10 seconds in duration) in a 7-hour study period.

V. Anesthetic considerations
A. Preoperative
1. Preoperative evaluation of morbidly obese patients should include a chest x-ray, EKG, arterial blood gas, and pulmonary function tests.
2. The airway should be carefully examined since these patients are often difficult to intubate as a result of limited mobility of the temporomandibular and atlanto-occipital joints, a narrowed upper airway, and a shortened distance between the mandible and sternal fat pads.
3. All obese patients are at an increased risk of aspiration and should be considered to have a full-stomach. Pretreatment with H_2 antagonists (both the night before and the morning of surgery), metoclopramide, and sodium citrate should be considered. Avoid sedation.

B. Intraoperative
1. The risk of rapid decreases in PaO_2 is significant; therefore, preoxygenation prior to intubation is essential.
2. Rapid sequence induction/intubation is selected to minimize the risk of pulmonary aspiration. Morbidly obese patients with a difficult airway should be intubated while awake.
3. Volatile anesthetics may be metabolized more extensively in obese patients. Obese patients are at an increased risk of halothane hepatitis.
4. Obese patients generally require 20-25% less local anesthetic for spinal or epidural anesthesia secondary to epidural fat and distended epidural veins.

C. Postoperative
1. Respiratory failure is the major postoperative problem of morbidly obese patients. Other problems include deep vein thrombosis, pulmonary embolism, and wound infections.
2. The semisitting position will optimize the mechanics of breathing (unload the diaphragm) and will minimize the development of arterial hypoxemia.

3. Patients generally should not be extubated until fully awake.

Liver Disease

I. **Preoperative evaluation and treatment**
   A. **Past medical history.** Evaluation of type of liver disease, previous or present jaundice, history of gastrointestinal bleeding; previous surgical operations; degree of ascites or encephalopathy should be noted.
   B. **Lab test.** CBC with platelet count, serum bilirubin, albumin, serum electrolytes (sodium, potassium, glucose), creatinine and BUN, PT/PTT, and liver function tests.
   C. **Preop LFTs.** Should be stable or decreasing for elective surgery.
   D. **Treatment**. The coagulation system function should be evaluated and corrected preoperatively (with vitamin K, FFP, or platelets as needed). Adequate hydration and diuresis (1 mL/kg/hr) should be achieved.
   E. **Premedications.** Sedatives should be omitted or the dose decreased.
II. **Halothane hepatic dysfunction**
   A. **Two entities**
      1. Mild/transient form related to hypoxia.
      2. Fulminant form possibly secondary to allergic reaction.
   B. Most often occurs in middle-aged obese females with recent exposure to halothane (up to 4 months). Halothane hepatic dysfunction manifest as post-operative fever and elevated liver function tests.
   C. Pediatric patients are less likely to have halothane-related hepatic dysfunction even after repeated exposures at short intervals.

Chemotherapy

1. **Cyclophosphamide (Cytoxan).** Myelosuppression, hemorrhagic cystitis, water retention, pulmonary fibrosis, plasma cholinesterase inhibition.
2. **Nitrogen Mustard.** Myelosuppression, local tissue damage.
3. **Vincristine.** Neurotoxicity, dilutional hyponatremia.
4. **Vinblastine.** Myelosuppression.
5. **Methotrexate.** Renal tubular injury.
6. **5-Fluorouracil and ARA C.** Hemorrhage enteritis, diarrhea, myelosuppression.
7. **Adriamycin.** Cardiac toxicity; risk factors include total cumulative dose over 550 mg/m2, concomitant cyclophosphamide therapy, prior history of heart disease, age over 65 years.
8. **Bleomycin.** Pulmonary toxicity; risk factors include total cumulative dose over 200 mg, concomitant thoracic radiation therapy, age over 65 years.
9. **Mitomycin C.** pulmonary toxicity.
10. **Cisplatin.** renal toxicity, neurotoxicity.
11. **Nitrosoureas (BCNU, CCNU).** myelosuppression, renal pulmonary toxicity.

26 Chemotherapy

12. **Taxol.** hypersensitivity reaction, myelosuppression, cardiac toxicity, peripheral neuropathy.
13. **Growth factors.** pulmonary edema, pericardial and pleural effusions.

Basics of Anesthesiology

Medical Gas Systems

I. **Oxygen**
   A. Oxygen is stored as a compressed gas at room temperature or refrigerated as a liquid.
   B. The pressure in an oxygen cylinder is directly proportional to the volume of oxygen in the cylinder.

II. **Nitrous oxide**
   A. At room temperature, nitrous oxide is stored as a liquid.
   B. In contrast to oxygen, the cylinder pressure for nitrous oxide does not indicate the amount of gas remaining in the cylinder. Cylinder pressure remains at 750 psi as long as any liquid nitrous oxide is present (when cylinder pressure begins to fall, only about 400 liters of nitrous oxide remains).
   C. The only way to determine residual volume of nitrous oxide is to weigh the cylinder.

Characteristics of Medical Gas Cylinders

	Oxygen	Nitrous Oxide	Carbon Dioxide	Air	Nitrogen
Cylinder Color	Green	Blue	Gray	Yellow	Black
Form	Gas	Liquid	Liquid	Gas	Gas
Capacity (L)	625	1590	1590	624	625
Pressure (psi)	2000	750	838	1800	2000

Electrical Safety

I. **Line isolation monitor**
   A. Line isolation monitor measures the potential for current flow from the isolated power supply to ground.
   B. An alarm is activated if an unacceptably high current flow to ground becomes possible (usually 2 mA or 5 mA).
   C. Operating room power supply is isolated from grounds by an isolation transformer. The line source is grounded by the electrical provider while the secondary circuit is intentionally not grounded.

II. **Electrical shock**
   A. Macroshock
      1. Macroshock refers to the application of electrical current through intact

skin.
   2. Currents exceeding 100 mA may result in VF.
  B. **Microshock**
   1. Microshock refers to the application of electrical current directly to the heart (ie, guide wires or pacing wires).
   2. Currents exceeding 50 microamps through a ventricular catheter may induce ventricular fibrillation.
   3. The national code requires less than 10 microamps maximum permissible leakage through electrodes or catheters that contact the heart. Line isolation monitors do not protect a patient from microshock.

Anesthesia Machine

I. **Safety valves and regulators**
  A. **Outlet check value.** Prevents gas cylinders from crossfilling.
  B. **Pressure regulator.** Reduces cylinder gas pressure to below 50 psi.
  C. **Fail-safe valve.** Closes nitrous oxide and other gas lines if oxygen pressure falls below 25 psi to prevent accidental delivery of a hypoxic mixture.
  D. **Diameter index safety system (DISS).** Prevents incorrect gas line attachment to the anesthesia machine.
  E. **Pin index safety system (PISS).** Interlink between the anesthesia machine and gas cylinder; prevents incorrect cylinder attachment.
  F. **Second stage oxygen pressure regulator.** Oxygen flow is constant until oxygen pressure drops below 12-16 PSI; whereas other gases shut off if oxygen pressure is less than 30 PSI. This ensures that oxygen is last gas flowing.
II. **Flowmeters** on anesthesia machines are classified as constant-pressure, variable orifice flowmeters.
III. **Vaporizers**
  A. **Classification of modern vaporizers**
   1. **Variable bypass.** Part of the total gas flow coming into the vaporizer is bypassed into the vaporizing chamber and then returns to join the rest of the gas at the outlet.
   2. **Flow-over.** The gas channeled to the vaporizing chamber flows over the liquid agent and becomes saturated.
   3. **Temperature-compensated.** Automatic temperature compensation device helps maintain a constant vaporizer output over a wide range of temperatures.
   4. **Agent specific.**
   5. **Out of circuit.** Not in the breathing circuit.
  B. **Vaporizer output** is not influenced by fresh gas flows until very low flow rates (<250 mL/min) or very high flow rates (>15 l/min).
IV. **Anesthesia ventilators**
  A. **Power source.** Contemporary ventilators have a pneumatic and electrical power source.
  B. **Drive mechanism.** Compressed gas is the driving mechanism.

Basics of Anesthesia 29

- **C. Cycling mechanism.** Time-cycled, and inspiration is triggered by a timing device.
- **D. Bellows classification.** Direction of the bellows during expiration determines the classification. Ascending bellows (bellow ascends during expiration) is safer; a ascending bellow will not fill if a disconnect occurs.
- **E.** Because the ventilator's pressure relief valve is closed during inspiration, the circuit's fresh gas flows contribute to the tidal volume delivered to the patient. The amount each tidal volume will increase. (fresh gas flow mL/min) x (% inspiratory time) divided by the respiratory rate.
- **F.** The use of the oxygen flush valve during the inspiratory cycle of a ventilator must be avoided because the pressure-relief valve is closed and the surge of circuit pressure will be transferred to the patient's lungs.

Patient Monitors

I. Capnogram
  A. The normal end-tidal to arterial CO_2 gradient (dCO_2) is 2-5 mmHg. This value reflects alveolar dead space (alveoli ventilated but not perfused).

  B. Causes of increased dCO_2.
  1. Decreased pulmonary arterial pressure.
  2. Upright posture.
  3. Pulmonary embolism. air, fat, thrombus, amniotic fluid.
  4. COPD: causes nonvascular air space at the alveolar level.
  5. Mechanical obstruction of the pulmonary arteries.
  6. Ventilation gas leaving the normal air passages. bronchopleural fistula, tracheal disruption, cuff leak.

  C. Causes of increased end-tidal CO_2
  1. Hypoventilation.
  2. Sodium bicarbonate.
  3. Laparoscopy (CO_2 inflation).
  4. Anesthetic breathing circuit error
     - a. Inadequate fresh gas flow.
     - b. Rebreathing.
     - c. Faulty circle absorber valves.
     - d. Exhausted soda lime.
  5. Hyperthermia.
  6. Improved blood flow to lungs following lung resuscitation or after hypotension.
  7. Water in capnograph head.

  D. Causes of decreased end-tidal CO_2
  1. Hyperventilation.
  2. Inadequate sampling volume.
  3. Incorrect placement of sampling catheter.
  4. Hypothermia.
  5. Incipient pulmonary edema.
  6. Air embolism.
  7. Decreased blood flow to lungs.

II. Pulse oximetry

A. Oxyhemoglobin absorbs more infrared light (eg, 660 nm), while deoxyhemoglobin absorbs more red light (eg, 940 nm).

B. The change in light absorption during arterial pulsations is the basis of oximetry determination of oxygen saturation.

C. Oxygen saturation of 90% indicates a PaO_2 of approximately 60 mmHg in normal adults.

D. Pulse oximeters that only compare two wavelengths of light will register a falsely high reading in patients with carbon monoxide poisoning because carboxyhemoglobin and oxyhemoglobin absorb light at 660 nm identically.

E. Methemoglobin has the same absorption coefficient at both red and infrared wavelengths, resulting in a 1:1 absorption ratio corresponding to a saturation reading of 85%. Thus, methemoglobinemia causes a falsely low saturation reading when SaO_2 is actually greater then 85% and a falsely high reading if SaO_2 is actually less than 85%.

F. Fetal hemoglobin and bilirubin do not affect pulse oximeter.

G. **Sources of error**
   1. **Dyshemoglobins**
      a. **Carboxyhemoglobin.** Because carboxyhemoglobin and oxyhemoglobin absorb light at 660 nm identically, pulse oximeters that only compare two wavelengths of light will register a falsely high reading in patients suffering from carbon monoxide poisoning.
      b. **Methemoglobin.** Methemoglobin has the same absorption coefficient at both red and infrared wavelengths, resulting in a 1:1 absorption ratio corresponding to a saturation reading of 85%. Thus, methemoglobinemia causes a falsely low saturation reading when SaO_2 is actually greater then 85% and a falsely high reading if SaO_2 is actually less than 85%.
   2. **Intravenous dyes**
      a. **Methylene blue.** Can cause large, rapid decrease in saturation without decreases in the actual oxygen saturation.
      b. **Indocyanine green**. Causes smaller false decreases in saturation.
      c. **IV fluorescein or indigo carmine** have little effect.
   3. **Excessive ambient light**. In cases of reduced pulse amplitude, pulse oximeters may become sensitive to external light sources, such as fluorescent room lights.
   4. **Motion artifact.**
   5. **Venous pulsations.** Pulse oximeter design assumes that the pulsatile component of the light absorbance is due to arterial blood.
   6. **Low perfusion.**
   7. **Leakage of light** from the light-emitting diode to the photodiode, bypassing the arterial bed.
   8. **Penumbra effect.** Pulse oximeters whose sensors are malpositioned may display SaO_2 values in the 90-95 per cent range on normoxemic subjects. This so-called "penumbra effect" can cause underestimation at high saturations, overestimation at low saturations, and a strong dependence of the error on instrument and sensor.

Anesthesia Machine Check

The anesthesia machine check list should be conducted before administering anesthesia.

I. Emergency ventilation equipment*
   A. Verify jet ventilator is hooked up and working.

II. Overview*
   A. Inspect machine for the following
   1. Plugged in.
   2. Flowmeters off.
   3. Vaporizers filled and caps tight.
   4. Tanks on machine properly.
   5. No obvious problems.
   6. Breathing circuit attached.

III. Electrical systems*
   A. Turn on master switch.
   B. Perform battery check.
   C. Turn on all monitors.

IV. High pressure systems*
   A. Check Oxygen cylinders
   1. Disconnect wall pipeline.
   2. Open O_2 tank.
   3. Open O_2 flowmeter.
   4. Tank should stay at least 1000 psi.
   5. Close tank.
   6. Low O_2 pressure alarm should respond as bobbin falls.
   7. Turn off O_2 flowmeter.
   8. Reconnect pipeline O_2.

   B. Check pipeline pressures (should read around 50 p.s.i.).

V. Low pressure systems*
   A. Test flowmeters
   1. Adjust flow of gases through their full range, checking for smooth operation.
   2. Check N_2O/O_2 ratio alarm by trying to create a hypoxic mixture (the gas switch should be set for "N_2O/O_2") and verify correct changes in flow.

   B. Check for low pressure leaks
   1. **Drager system** (no back-check valve)
      a. Turn O_2 flowmeter to 400 cc/min.
      b. Open vaporizer.
      c. Occlude gas outlet. bobbin should fall.
      d. Open gas outlet. bobbin should rise.
      e. Close vaporizer.
   2. **Ohmeda system** (back-check valve)
      a. Turn of master switch and flowmeters.
      b. Attach suction bulb to common gas outlet.
      c. Squeeze bulb repeatedly until it collapses.
      d. Verify that bulb stays collapsed for 10 seconds.
      e. Repeat with vaporizers turned on.

32 Anesthesia Machine Check

      f. Turn on switch and turn off vaporizers.
VI. Scavenging system*
A. Adjust and check scavenging system
1. Ensure proper connections between scavenging system and both APL (popoff valve) and the ventilator relief valve.
2. Close scavenge valve, then open 1½ turns.
3. Fully open APL valve and occlude the Y-piece.
4. With minimum O_2 flow, scavenger reservoir should collapse completely. Verify that PIP valve reads zero (checks negative pressure valve).
5. With O_2 flush activated, allow the scavenger reservoir bag to distend fully and check that PIP valve reads less than 10 cm/H_2O (checks positive pressure pop-off valve).

VII. Breathing system
A. Calibrate O_2 monitor*
1. Ensure monitor reads 21% room air.
2. Verify that low O_2 alarm is enabled and functioning.
3. Reinstall sensor in circuit and flush breathing system with 100% oxygen
4. Verify that monitor now reads greater than 90%.

B. Check initial status of system
1. Set selector switch to "bag" mode.
2. Check that breathing circuit is complete, undamaged, and unobstructed.
3. Verify that CO_2 absorbent is adequate.
4. Install any accessory equipment such as humidifier.

C. Perform leak check of breathing circuit
1. Set all gas flows to minimum.
2. Close APL valve and occlude Y piece.
3. Pressurize breathing system to 30 cm H_2O with O_2 flush.
4. Ensure that pressure remains fixed for at least 10 seconds.
5. Open APL valve and ensure that pressure decreases.

VIII. Manual and automatic ventilation systems
A. Test ventilation systems and unidirectional valves
1. Set appropriate tidal volume (TV), rate, inspiratory flow.
2. Make sure PEEP valve is off.
3. Set to ventilator mode.
4. Place breathing bag on Y-piece.
5. Turn ventilator on and fill bellows with O_2 flush valve.
6. Set O_2 to minimum and other gas flows to "0".
7. Verify that, during inspiration, bellow delivers appropriate TV and that bellows empties completely on expiration.
8. Set fresh gas flow to about 5 liters per minute.
9. Verify that the ventilator bellows and simulated lungs fill and empty appropriately without sustained pressure at end expiration.
10. Check for proper action of unidirectional valves.
11. Turn ventilator off and switch to manual ventilation.
12. Ventilate manually and assure inflation and deflation of artificial lungs

IX. Monitors
A. Check, calibrate, and/or set alarm limits of all monitors
1. Capnometer and respiratory volume monitor.
2. O_2 analyzer.
3. Pulse oximeter.
4. Set-up and calibrate invasive monitor transducers.
5. Airway pressure high and low alarms.
6. Automatic BP cuff.
7. EKG monitor.
8. Temperature probe available.
9. Transcutaneous O_2.

X. Final check
A. Check final status of machine
1. Vaporizers off.
2. APL open.
3. Selector switch should be set to "bag".
4. All flowmeters should be zero (O_2 to minimum flow).
5. Patient suction level adequate.
6. Breathing system ready to use.

XI. Additional equipment if needed*
1. Blood warmers/Level 1.
2. Bear Hugger.
3. Warming blanket.
4. Operating room table works.
5. Portable oxygen available.

*These steps need not be repeated if same provider uses the machine in successive cases

Pharmacology

Basic Pharmacology

I. Stages of general anesthesia
  A. **Stage 1 (amnesia)** begins with induction of anesthesia and ends with the loss of consciousness (loss of eyelid reflex). Pain perception threshold during this stage is not lowered.
  B. **Stage 2 (delirium/excitement)** is characterized by uninhibited excitation. Agitation, delirium, irregular respiration and breath holding. Pupils are dilated and eyes are divergent. Responses to noxious stimuli can occur during this stage may include vomiting, laryngospasm, hypertension, tachycardia, and uncontrolled movement.
  C. **Stage 3 (surgical anesthesia)** is characterized by central gaze, constricted pupils, and regular respirations. Target depth of anesthesia is sufficient when painful stimulation does not elicit somatic reflexes or deleterious autonomic responses.
  D. **Stage 4 (impending death/overdose)** is characterized by onset of apnea, dilated and nonreactive pupils, and hypotension to complete failure of the circulation.

II. Components of general anesthesia
  A. Unconsciousness (hypnosis).
  B. Analgesia (areflexia).
  C. Muscle relaxation.

III. Pharmacokinetics of inhaled anesthetics
  A. **Anesthetic concentration.** The fraction of a gas in a mixture is equal to the volume of that gas divided by the total volume of the mixture.
  B. **Partial pressure.** The partial pressure of a component gas in a mixture is equal to the fraction it contributes toward total pressure.
  C. **Minimum alveolar concentration (MAC)**
  1. The minimum alveolar concentration of an inhalation agent is the minimum concentration necessary to prevent movement in 50% of patients in response to a surgical skin incision.
  2. The minimum alveolar concentrations required to prevent eye opening on verbal command, to prevent movement and coughing in response to endotracheal intubation, and to prevent adrenergic response to skin incision have been defined. These are called MAC Awake, MAC Endotracheal Intubation, and MAC BAR (for blockade of autonomic response). In general, MAC Awake is 50% MAC, MAC Endotracheal Intubation is 130% MAC, and MAC BAR is 150% MAC. MAC Amnesia, 25% MAC, has defined as the concentration that blocks anterograde memory in 50% of awake patients.
  3. MAC values for different volatile agents are additive. The lower the MAC the more potent the agent.
  4. The highest MACs are found in infants at term to 6 months of age. The MAC decreases with both increasing age and prematurity.
  5. Factors that increase MAC include hyperthermia, drugs that increase

CNS catecholamines, infants, hypernatremia, and chronic ethanol abuse.
6. Factors that decrease MAC include hypothermia (for every Celsius degree drop in body temperature, MAC decreases 2-5%), preoperative medications, IV anesthetics, neonates, elderly, pregnancy, alpha-2 agonists, acute ethanol ingestion, lithium, cardiopulmonary bypass, opioids, and PaO_2 less than 38 mmHg.
7. Factors that have no effect on MAC include duration of anesthesia, gender, thyroid gland dysfunction, hyperkalemia, and hypokalemia.

D. **Alveolar uptake.** The rate of alveolar uptake is determined by the following factors:
1. **Inspired concentration.** A high inspired anesthetic partial pressure (PI) accelerates induction of anesthesia. This effect of the high PI is known as the concentration effect.
2. **Alveolar ventilation.** Increased ventilation increases the rate of alveolar uptake of anesthetic. The net effect is a more rapid rate of rise in the alveolar partial pressure of an inhaled anesthetic and induction of anesthesia.
3. **Anesthetic breathing system.** The rate of rise of the alveolar partial pressure of an inhaled anesthetic is influenced by (1) the volume of the system, (2) solubility of the inhaled anesthetics into the components of the system, and (3) gas inflow from the anesthetic machine.
4. **Uptake of the inhaled anesthetic**
   a. **Solubility.** The solubility of inhaled anesthetics is defined as the amount of anesthetic agent required to saturate a unit volume of blood at a given temperature and can be expressed as the blood:gas partition coefficient. The more soluble the agent, the greater the uptake into the pulmonary capillaries. The solubility of the inhalation agent in blood is the most important single factor in determining the speed of induction and recovery in individual patients.
   b. **Cardiac output.** A high cardiac output results in more rapid uptake such that the rate of rise in the alveolar partial pressure and the speed of induction are slowed.
   c. **Alveolar to venous partial pressure difference.** A large alveolar to venous gradient enhances the uptake of anesthetic by pulmonary blood and tends to slow the rise in the alveolar partial pressure.

E. **Second gas effect.** The ability of the large volume uptake of one gas (first gas) to accelerate the rate of rise of the alveolar partial pressure of a concurrently administered companion gas (second gas) is known as the second gas effect.

F. **Elimination.** Most of the inhaled agents are exhaled unchanged by the lungs. Hyperventilation, a small FRC (function residual capacity), a low solubility, a low cardiac output, or a large mixed venous-alveolar tension gradient increases the rate of decay.

G. **Diffusion hypoxia** results from dilution of alveolar oxygen concentration by the large amount of nitrous oxide leaving the pulmonary capillary blood at the conclusion of nitrous oxide administration. This can be prevented by filling the patient's lungs with oxygen at the conclusion of nitrous oxide administration.

IV. Pharmacokinetics of intravenous anesthetics

A. Volume of distribution.
The apparent volume into which a drug has been distributed is called the volume of distribution. The volume of distribution reflects the volume of plasma that would be necessary to account for the observed plasma concentration.

B. Plasma concentration curves
1. **Distribution (alpha) phase.** The alpha phase corresponds to the initial distribution of drug from the circulation to tissues.
2. **Elimination (beta) phase.** The second phase is characterized by a gradual decline in the plasma concentration of drug and reflects its elimination from the central vascular compartment by renal and hepatic mechanisms.

C. Elimination half-time
is the time necessary for the plasma concentration of drug to decline 50 percent during the elimination phase.

D. Physical characteristics of the drug
1. Highly lipid-soluble drugs (most intravenous anesthetics) are taken up rapidly by tissues.
2. With water soluble agents, molecular size is an important determinant of diffusibility across plasma membranes.
3. Degree of ionization. the degree of ionization is determined by the pH of the biophase and the pKa of the drug. Only nonionized (basic) molecules diffuse across the biological membranes.

Local Anesthetics

I. Mechanism of action of local anesthetics
A. Local anesthetics prevent increases in neural membrane permeability to sodium ions, slowing the rate of depolarization so that threshold potential is never reached and no action potential is propagated.
B. Local anesthetics gain access to sodium channels only when they are in their activated state. Rapidly firing nerves are more sensitive and, therefore, are blocked first.

II. Metabolism

A. Esters
1. Ester local anesthetics are predominantly metabolized by pseudocholinesterase (plasma cholinesterase). Cerebrospinal fluid lacks esterase enzymes, so the termination of action of intrathecally injected ester local anesthetics depends upon their absorption into the bloodstream
2. P-aminobenzoic acid, a metabolite of local anesthetics, has been associated with allergic reactions.

B. Amides
1. Metabolized by microsomal enzymes in the liver.
2. Metabolites of prilocaine (o-toluidine derivatives), which accumulate

after large doses (greater than 10 mg/kg), convert hemoglobin to methemoglobin. Other drugs that can cause methemoglobinemia include benzocaine.

III. Physiochemical factors

A. Lipid solubility. Increased lipid solubility increases potency.

B. Protein binding. The greater the protein binding, the longer the duration of action.

C. pKa determines the onset time. The closer the pKa of the local anesthetic is to tissue pH, the greater the fraction of the non-ionized, lipid-soluble form, is available, and the faster the onset.

D. Ion trapping. Refers to the accumulation of the ionized form of a local anesthetic in acidic environments due to a pH gradient between the ionized and non-ionized forms. This can occur between a mother and an acidotic fetus (ie, fetal distress), resulting in the accumulation of local anesthetic in fetal blood.

E. Minimum concentration of local anesthetic (Cm) is the minimum concentration of local anesthetic that will block nerve impulse conduction and is analogous to the minimum alveolar concentration (MAC) of inhalation anesthetics.

IV. Rate of systemic absorption of local anesthetics (from high to low).

Intravenous > tracheal > intercostal > caudal > paracervical > epidural > brachial plexus > sciatic/femoral > subcutaneous.

V. Uses of local anesthetics

A. Topical. Lidocaine, cocaine, tetracaine.

B. Infiltration. Lidocaine, bupivacaine, procaine, chloroprocaine, mepivacaine, etidocaine, prilocaine.

C. Peripheral nerve block. Lidocaine, bupivacaine, procaine, chloroprocaine, mepivacaine, etidocaine, prilocaine.

D. IV regional. Lidocaine, bupivacaine, prilocaine.

E. Epidural. Lidocaine, chloroprocaine, bupivacaine, prilocaine, etidocaine, mepivacaine.

F. Spinal. Lidocaine, tetracaine, procaine, bupivacaine.

VI. Adjuvants

A. Epinephrine may be added to local anesthetics to produce local vasoconstriction, limiting systemic absorption, prolonging duration of effect, and decreasing surgical bleeding

B. The maximum dose of epinephrine should not exceed 10 mcg/kg in pediatric patients and 200-250 mcg in adults.

C. Adding sodium bicarbonate raises the pH and increases the concentration of nonionized free base. 1 mEq of sodium bicarbonate is added to each 10 cc of lidocaine.

VII. Effects of local anesthetics on organ systems

A. Cardiac

1. Local anesthetics depress myocardial automaticity (spontaneous phase IV depolarization) and reduce the duration of the refractory period.
2. Cardiac dysrhythmia or circulatory collapse is often a presenting sign of local anesthetic overdose during general anesthesia.

3. Intravascular injection of bupivacaine has produced severe cardiotoxic reactions, including hypotension, atrioventricular heart block, and dysrhythmias such as ventricular fibrillation. Pregnancy, hypoxemia, and respiratory acidosis are predisposing risk factors.

B. Respiratory Effects
1. Lidocaine depresses the hypoxic drive (the ventilatory response to low PaO_2).
2. Apnea can result from phrenic and intercostal nerve paralysis or depression of the medullary respiratory center following direct exposure to local anesthetic agents (eg, postretrobulbar apnea syndrome).

C. Cerebral Effects
1. Early symptoms of overdose include circumoral numbness, tongue paresthesia, and dizziness. Sensory complaints may include tinnitus and burred vision. Excitatory signs (eg, restlessness, agitation, nervousness, paranoia) often precede central nervous system depression (slurred speech, drowsiness, unconsciousness).
2. Tonic-clonic seizures may result from selective blockade of inhibitory pathways. Respiratory arrest often follows seizure activity.
3. **Neurotoxicity**
   a. Chloroprocaine has been associated with neurotoxicity. The cause of this neural toxicity may be the low pH of chloroprocaine (pH 3.0).
   b. Repeated doses of 5% lidocaine and 0.5% tetracaine have been associated with neurotoxicity (cauda equina syndrome) following infusion through small-bore catheters used in continuous spinal anesthesia. This may be due to pooling of drug around the cauda equina.

D. Immunologic Effects
1. Allergic or hypersensitivity reactions are very rare with local anesthetics. Esters are more likely to induce an allergic reaction because they are derivatives of p-aminobenzoic acid, a known allergen.
2. Allergic reactions to amides are extremely rare and are probably related to the preservative and not the amide itself. Multidose preparations of amides often contain methylparaben, which has a chemical structure similar to that of p-aminobenzoic acid.

E. Musculoskeletal Effects.
Local anesthetics are myotoxic when injected directly into skeletal muscle.

F. Neurotoxicity.
5% lidocaine as been implicated in of cauda-equina syndrome. 1.5% lidocaine with dextrose or preservative free 2% lidocaine is recommended.

Local Anesthetics: Dosages For Infiltration Anesthesia

	Plain Solution		Epinephrine Solution	
Drug	Max Dose (mg)	Duration (min)	Max Dose (mg)	Duration (min)
Procaine	400	30-60	600	
Chloroprocaine	800	30-45	1000	30-90
Lidocaine	300	30-120	500	120-360
Mepivacaine	300	45-90	500	120-360
Prilocaine	500	30-90	600	120-360
Bupivacaine	175	120-240	225	180-420
Etidocaine	300	120-180	400	180-420

Local Anesthetics: Dosages For Spinal Anesthesia

Drug	Concentration (%)	T10 Level (mg)	T6 Level (mg)	T4 Level (mg)	Duration Plain (min)	Duration w/epi (min)
Procaine	10	75	125	200	30-45	60-75
Lidocaine	5.0	25	50-75	75-100	45-60	60-90
Tetracaine*	0.5**	6-8	8-14	14-20	60-90	120-180
Bupivacaine	0.75	4-6	8-12	12-20	120-150	120-150

*For hypobaric spinal: tetracaine diluted with sterile water to 0.3% solution
**Preparation concentration of tetracaine is 1%; tetracaine is diluted with 5.0% glucose for hyperbaric solution and normal saline for isobaric solution

Local Anesthetics: Dosages For Epidural Anesthesia

Drug	Usual Conc %	Usual Vol (mL)	Total Dose (mg)	Onset (min)	Duration (min)
Chloroprocaine	2-3	15-30	300-900	5-15	30-90
Lidocaine	1-2	15-30	150-500	5-15	60-120
Mepivacaine	1-2	15-30	150-300	5-15	60-180
Prilocaine	1-3	15-30	150-600	5-15	60-180

40 Pharmacology

Bupivacaine	0.25-0.75	25-30	37.5-225	5-15	120-240
Etidocaine	1.0-1.5	15-30	150-300	5-15	120-240

Local Anesthetics: Maximum Dose

Drug	Plain (mg)	Epi (mg)	Plain (mg/kg)	Epi (mg/kg)
Amides				
Bupivacaine	175	225	3	
Dibucaine			1	
Etidocaine	300	400	4	
Lidocaine	300	500	4.5	7
Mepivacaine	300	500	4.5	7
Prilocaine	400		8	
Esters				
Chloroprocaine	600	1000	12	
Cocaine			3	
Procaine	500	600	12	
Tetracaine	100	200	3	

Muscle Relaxants

Drug	ED 95 (mg/kg)	Onset (min)	Duration (min)	Histamine Release	Elimination And Misc
Succinyl-choline	0.25	1	5-10	Rare	Plasma cholinesterase, muscarinic and nicotinic stim
d-Tubo-curarine	0.51	3-5	60-90	+++	70% renal; 20% biliary; autonomic ganglia block
Metocurine	0.28	3-5	60-90	++	80-100% renal; autonomic ganglia blockade
Pancuronium	0.07	3-5	60-90	None	70% renal; 15-20% liver; muscarinic block
Pipecuronium	0.07	3-5	60-90	None	
Doxacurium	0.25-0.4	4-6	60-90	None	35% renal
Atracurium	0.20	3-5	20-35	+	Hofmann elim & ester hydrolysis, laudanosine

Pharmacology

Cis-atracurium	0.05	1-2	60	None	Hofmann elimination
Vecuronium	0.05	3-5	20-35	None	10-20% renal; 40-60% biliary; 20% hepatic
Mivacurium	0.08	2-3	12-20	+	plasma cholinesterase
Gallamine	2.5	4-5	70-80	None	80-100% renal; muscarinic block
Rocuronium	0.3	1-2	20-35	None	10-25% renal; 50-70% biliary; 10-20% hepatic

Dosages of Muscle Relaxants

	Sup Dose(mg/kg)			Infusions (mcg/kg/min)		
Drug	Intubate Dose (mg/kg)	N₂O/ Opioid	Inhalation	Load Dose (mg/kg)	N₂O/ Opioid	Inhalation
Succinylcholine	1.0-1.5			1.0-1.5	60-100	30-50
d-Tubocurarine	0.6	0.1	0.05			
Metocurine	0.4	0.07	0.04			
Pancuronium	0.1	0.015	0.007			
Pipecuronium	0.14					
Doxacurium	0.05-0.08	0.005-0.025				
Atracurium	0.4-0.5	0.1	0.07	0.3-0.5	5-10	3-6
Cis-atracurium	0.15-0.2	0.03			1-2	
Vecuronium	0.08-0.1	0.02	0.015	0.06-0.1	1-2	0.6-1.2
Mivacurium	0.15-0.25*	0.1	0.1		5-10	
Rocuronium	0.6-1.2	0.075-0.15			6-10	

*Given in divided doses (0.15 mg/kg followed in 30 seconds by 0.10 mg/kg). For children 2 to 12 years of age, the recommended dose of mivacurium is 0.20 mg/kg, administered over 5 to 15 seconds.

Neuromuscular Blocking Agents

I. Depolarizing blockade
A. Succinylcholine is the only depolarizing muscle relaxant that is made up of two joined acetylcholine molecules. Succinylcholine mimics the action of acetylcholine by depolarizing the postsynaptic membrane at the neuromuscular junction.
B. Metabolism
1. Rapid onset of action (30-60 seconds) with a short duration of action (5-10 minutes).
2. Succinylcholine is rapidly metabolized by pseudocholinesterase into succinylmonocholine so that only a fraction (approximately 10%) of the injected does ever reaches the neuromuscular junction.
3. As serum levels fall, succinylcholine molecules diffuse away from the neuromuscular junction.

C. Adverse side effects of succinylcholine
1. **Cardiac.** Sinus bradycardia, junctional rhythm, sinus arrest. Ganglionic stimulation may increase heart rate and blood pressure in adults. Succinylcholine may produce bradycardia in children after first dose and after second dose in adults.
2. **Hyperkalemia**
   a. Normal muscle releases enough potassium during succinylcholine-induced depolarization to raise serum potassium by 0.5 mEq/L.
   b. Massive release of intracellular potassium can result from situations where there is a proliferation of extrajunctional receptors. Conditions associated with succinylcholine-induced hyperkalemia include: patients with thermal injuries, massive trauma, severe intra-abdominal infection, neurologic disorders (spinal cord injury, encephalitis, stroke, Guillain-Barre syndrome, severe Parkinson's disease), ruptured cerebral aneurysm, polyneuropathy, myopathies (eg, Duchenne's dystrophy) and tetanus. This potassium release is not reliably prevented by pretreatment with a nondepolarizer muscle relaxant.
3. **Increased intracranial pressure.** Increased cerebral blood flow, and increased intraocular pressure
4. **Increased intragastric pressure.** The increase in intragastric pressure is offset by an increase in lower esophageal sphincter tone.
5. **Myalgia** and myoglobinuria.
6. **Fasciculations.** Can be prevented by pretreatment with a small dose of nondepolarizing relaxant.
7. **Trismus.** Patients afflicted with myotonia may develop myoclonus after succinylcholine administration.
8. **Malignant hyperthermia**.
9. **Phase II block** may occur with repeated or continuous infusions and is characterized by tetanic or TOF fade, tachyphylaxis, partial or complete reversal with anticholinesterases.
10. **Prolonged Blockade**
    a. Decreased plasma cholinesterase in last trimester of pregnancy, liver disease, starvation, carcinomas, hypothyroidism, burn patients, and cardiac failure.

- **b.** Inhibition of plasma cholinesterase.
- **c.** Plasma cholinesterase deficiency.

D. Pseudocholinesterase abnormalities
1. Heterozygous atypical enzyme. 1 in 50 patients has one normal and one abnormal gene, resulting in a prolonged block (20-30 minutes).
2. Homozygous atypical enzyme: 1 in 3000 patients has two abnormal genes, which produce an enzyme with 1/100 the normal affinity for succinylcholine. Blockade may last 6-8 hours or longer.
3. Dibucaine, a local anesthetic, inhibits normal pseudocholinesterase activity by 80%, but inhibits the homozygous atypical enzyme by only 20% and the heterozygous enzyme by 40-60%. The percentage of inhibition of pseudocholinesterase activity is termed the dibucaine number. The dibucaine number is proportional to pseudocholinesterase function and independent of the amount of enzyme.

E. Drug interactions with succinylcholine
1. Cholinesterase inhibitors enhance the action of succinylcholine. Echothiophate eye drops and organophosphate pesticides fall into this category.
2. Nondepolarizing muscle relaxants antagonize depolarizing phase I blocks. An exception to this interaction is pancuronium, which augments succinylcholine blockade by inhibiting pseudocholinesterase.
3. Other drugs (that potentiate the neuromuscular block) include antibiotics (streptomycins, colistin, polymyxin, tetracycline, lincomycin, clindamycin), antidysrhythmics (quinidine, lidocaine, calcium channel blockers), antihypertensives (trimethaphan), cholinesterase inhibitors, furosemide, inhalational anesthetics, local anesthetics, lithium, and magnesium.

II. Non-depolarizing neuromuscular agents.
Drugs that potentiate nondepolarizing relaxants volatile agents, local anesthetics, calcium channel blockers, aminoglycosides, polymyxins, lincosamines, hexamethonium, trimethaphan, immunosuppressants, high-dose benzodiazepines, dantrolene, and magnesium.

III. Sensitivity to neuromuscular blockade.
Muscles have different sensitivities to muscle relaxants. The most resistant to most sensitive muscles are: vocal cord, diaphragm, orbicularis oculi, abdominal rectus, adductor pollicis, masseter, pharyngeal, extraocular.

IV. Common sites of neurostimulation
include the ulnar, posterior tibial, peroneal and facial nerves.

Comparison of Tests of Neuromuscular Function

Test	Estimated Receptors Occupied (%)
Tidal volume	80
Twitch height	75-80
Tetanic stimulation (30 Hz)	75-80
Vital capacity	75-80

Train-of-four	75-80
Tetanic stimulation (100 Hz)	50
Inspiratory force	50
Head lift (5 seconds)	33

Anticholinergics

I. **Mechanism of action.** Anticholinergics competitively block binding by acetylcholine and prevent receptor activation acetylcholine.
II. **Central anticholinergic syndrome**
   A. Scopolamine and atropine can enter the central nervous system and produce symptoms of restlessness and confusion that may progress to somnolence and unconsciousness. Other systemic manifestations include dry mouth, tachycardia, atropine flush, atropine fever, and impaired vision.
   B. Physostigmine, a tertiary amine anticholinesterase, is lipid-soluble and effectively reverses central anticholinergic toxicity. An initial dose of 0.01-0.03 mg/kg is recommended and may need to be repeated after 15-30 minutes.
   C. Glycopyrrolate does not easily cross the blood-brain barrier, and thus does not cause a central anticholinergic syndrome.

Pharmacological Characteristics of Anticholinergic Drugs			
	Atropine	Scopolamine	Glycopyrrolate
Tachycardia	+++	+	++
Bronchodilation	++	+	++
Sedation	+	+++	0
Antisialagogue	++	+++	++
Amnesia	+	+++	0

O = No effect; + = Minimal effect; ++ = Moderate effect; +++ = Marked effect

Anticholinesterases

	Edro-phonium	Neostigmine	Pyrido-stigmine	Physo-stigmine
Dose (mg/kg)	0.5-1.0	0.035-0.07 (up to 5 mg)	0.15-0.35	0.01-0.03
Onset (min)	Rapid (1)	Intermediate (7)	Delayed (10-13)	
Duration (min)	40-65	55-75	80-130	
Renal Excretion (%)	70	50	75	metabolized by plasma esterases
Atropine (mcg/kg)	7-10	15-30	15-20	usually not needed
Glycopyrrolate (mcg/kg)	do not use	7	7	

Muscarinic Side Effects of Cholinesterase Inhibitors

Organ System	Muscarinic Side Effect
Cardiovascular	Decreased heart rate, dysrhythmias
Pulmonary	Bronchospasm, increased bronchial secretions
Cerebral	Diffuse excitation (physostigmine only)
Gastrointestinal	Intestinal spasm, increased salivation
Genitourinary	Increased bladder tone
Ophthalmologic	Pupillary constriction

Benzodiazepines

I. Mechanism of action
  A. Benzodiazepines selectively attach to alpha subunits to enhance the chloride channel gating function of the inhibitory neurotransmitter GABA. Benzodiazepine receptors mostly occur on postsynaptic nerve endings in the central nervous system.

46 Pharmacology

Benzodiazepines

	Midazolam (Versed)	Diazepam (Valium)	Lorazepam (Ativan)
Relative Potency	3	1	5
Induction	0.15-0.35 mg/kg	0.3-0.5 mg/kg	0.1 mg/kg
Maintenance	0.05 mg/kg prn or 0.25-1.5 mcg/kg/min	0.1 mg/kg prn	0.02 mg/kg prn
Sedation	PO: 0.5-0.75 mg/kg IV: 0.025-0.1 mg/kg IM: 0.07-0.08 mg/kg PR: 0.3-0.35 mg/kg Nasal: 0.25-0.3 mg/kg	2 mg repeated	IV/IM: 0.02-0.08 mg/kg PO: 2-3 mg
Elimination Half-Time (h)	1-4	21-37	10-20

II. Cardiovascular effects
  A. Minimal cardiovascular effects.
  B. Midazolam tends to reduce blood pressure and peripheral vascular resistance more than diazepam.

III. Respiratory effects.
Depression of the ventilatory response to $PaCO_2$.

IV. Cerebral effects
  A. Reduced cerebral oxygen consumption, cerebral blood flow and ICP.
  B. Prevention and control of grand mal seizures.
  C. Mild muscle relaxation mediated at the spinal cord level.

V. Miscellaneous effects
  A. Benzodiazepines reduce MAC by up to 30%. Cimetidine reduces metabolism of diazepam.
  B. Pain during IV/IM injection and thrombophlebitis occurs with diazepam (secondary to its organic solvent propylene glycol).
  C. Erythromycin inhibits midazolam metabolism.
  D. Heparin displaces diazepam from protein binding sites and increases the free drug concentration.

VI. Reversal
  A. Benzodiazepines can be reversed by flumazenil (Romazicon). Flumazenil is a competitive inhibitor of GABA.
  B. For reversal of conscious sedation. 0.2 mg IV over 15 seconds. Give additional 0.1 mg IV bolus every 60 seconds to achieve desired effect, to a total of 1 mg. For reversal of overdose. 0.2 mg IV over 30 seconds. If necessary, give 0.3 mg IV 60 seconds later. If no effect, give 0.5 mg boluses every 60 seconds to a total of 3 mg. For reversal of resedation. 0.2 mg IV as required, to a total of 1 mg/hr, or infusion 0.5 mg/hr.
  C. Duration of antagonism is brief and may require repeated doses.
  D. Flumazenil may induce seizures, acute withdrawal, nausea, dizziness,

agitation, or arrhythmias (particularly in the presence of tricyclic antidepressants).

Opioids

I. **Classification of opioid receptors**
   A. **Mu receptor.** Morphine is the prototype exogenous ligand.
      1. **Mu-1.** The main action at this receptor is analgesia, but also responsible for miosis, nausea/vomiting, urinary retention, and pruritus. The endogenous ligands are enkephalins.
      2. **Mu-2.** Respiratory depression, euphoria, sedation, bradycardia, ileus and physical dependence are elicited by binding at this receptor.
   B. **Delta.** Modulation of mu receptor, physical dependence. High selective for the endogenous enkephalins, but opioid drugs still bind (leuenkephalin and beta-endorphin).
   C. **Kappa.** Ketocyclazocine and dynorphin are the prototype exogenous and endogenous ligands, respectively. Analgesia, sedation, dysphoria, and psychomimetic effects are produced by this receptor. Binding to the kappa receptor inhibits release of vasopressin and thus promotes diuresis. Pure kappa agonists do not produce respiratory depression.
   D. **Sigma.** N-allylnormetazocine is the prototype exogenous ligand. While this receptor binds many types of compounds, only levorotatory opioid isomers have opioid activity. The sigma receptor binds primarily dextrorotatory compounds. Dysphoria, hypertonia, tachycardia, tachypnea, and mydriasis are the principal effects of this receptor.

II. **Opioid systemic effects**
   A. **CNS.** CNS depression; pupillary constriction; nausea/vomiting (stimulates chemoreceptor trigger zone); hyperactive spinal reflexes; CNS excitation and seizures (high dose meperidine); analgesia; depressed cough reflex.
   B. **Cardiac.** Bradycardia (stimulation of vagal nucleus in medulla); tachycardia (meperidine); arteriolar and venous dilation (orthostatic hypotension); histamine release (morphine and meperidine); cardiac depression (meperidine).
   C. **Respiratory.** Increased arterial carbon dioxide tension; decreased breathing rate; increased tidal volume; decreased minute ventilation; decreased ventilatory response to carbon dioxide (CO_2 response curve moved to the right); chest wall rigidity.
   D. **Gastrointestinal.** Urinary retention; slow gastric emptying, spasm of sphincter of Oddi (less with meperidine).
   E. **Endocrine.** May block stress response to surgery at high doses.
   F. **Skeletal Muscle.** High doses may cause spasm of the thoracoabdominal muscles (chest wall rigidity).
   G. **Genitourinary tract.** Increases tone of ureter and vesicle sphincter, making voiding difficult (can be reversed with atropine).
   H. **Placenta.** can cross the placenta causing neonatal depression.
   I. **Drug interactions.** Administration of meperidine in a patient taking a monoamine oxidase inhibitor may result in delirium or hyperthermia.

III. Remifentanil (Ultiva)

A. Dosing

1. **General anesthesia.** An initial dose of 0.5-1 mcg/kg may be administered over 30-60 seconds if endotracheal intubation is to occur less than 8 minutes after the start of the infusion of remifentanil. Continuous infusion dose range is 0.05-2 mcg/kg/min, depending on which other agents are combined with remifentanil for maintenance anesthesia.
2. **Monitored anesthesia care (MAC).** May be administered as a single dose of 0.5-1.0 mcg/kg (over 30-60 seconds) 90 seconds prior to the placement of a local or regional anesthetic block.

B. Special considerations

1. **Muscle rigidity.** Remifentanil can cause muscle rigidity and is related to the dose and speed of administration. The occurrence of muscle rigidity is markedly reduced by administering hypnotics and/or a neuromuscular blocking agent prior to or in conjunction with remifentanil.
2. **Hypotension and bradycardia.** Both have been reported and respond to decreases in the administration of remifentanil, IV fluids or catecholamine administration.
3. **Rapid offset of action** occurs within 5-10 minutes after the discontinuation, no residual opioid activity will be present.

C. Special patient populations

1. **Pediatric patients.** No differences in pharmacokinetics are noted in children. The safety of remifentanil in children under the age of 2 years has not been established.
2. **Patients with renal or hepatic impairment.** No clinical differences are noted compared to healthy patients.
3. **Obese patients.** Dosing should be based on ideal, rather than actual, body weight in obese patients.
4. **Elderly patients.** Elderly patients are more sensitive to the effects of opioids; therefore, a 50% reduction in dose is recommended for elderly patients.

Opioids					
	Meperidine	Morphine	Fentanyl	Sufenta	Alfentanil
Equivalent Potency	0.1	1	75 to 125	500-1000	25
Rapid Distribution Half-Time (min)		1.2-2.5	1.4-1.7	1.4	1-3.5
Slow Distribution Half-Time (min)		9-13.3	13-28	17.7	8.2-16.8
Elimination Half-Time (min)	180-264	102-132	185-219	148-164	70-98
Clearance (mL/min/kg)	10-17	14.7	11.6	12.7	6.4
Vol of Distribution (l/kg)	2.8-4.2	3.2	4.1	2.86	0.86

	Meperidine	Morphine	Fentanyl	Sufenta	Alfentanil
Partition Coefficient (lipid solubility)			816	1727	129
Protein Binding (%)	60	26-36	79-87	92.5	89-92

Opioid Antagonist

I. Naloxone
A. Pure opioid antagonists. Administration results in displacement of opioid agonists from opioid receptors.
B. 1-4 mcg/kg IV will reverse opioid-induced analgesia and respiratory depression.
C. Continuous infusion, 5 mcg/kg/hr IV, will prevent respiratory depression without altering the analgesia produced by neuraxial opioids.
D. **Side effects.** Sudden antagonism can activate the sympathetic nervous system, resulting in cardiovascular stimulation.

Intravenous Induction Agents

I. Sodium thiopental (Pentothal) and other barbiturates
A. **Preparation.** A barbiturate; prepared as a 2.5% solution; water-soluble; pH of 10.5; stable for up to 1-2 weeks if refrigerated.
B. **Mechanism of action.** Depresses the reticular activating system, reflecting the ability of barbiturates to decrease the rate of dissociation of the inhibitory neurotransmitter gamma-aminobutyric acid from its receptors.
C. **Pharmacokinetics**
   1. Short duration of action (5-10 minutes) following IV bolus reflects high lipid solubility and redistribution from the brain to inactive tissues.
   2. Protein binding parallels lipid solubility, decreased protein binding increases drug sensitivity.
   3. Protein binding of thiopental in neonates is about half that in adults, suggesting a possible increased sensitivity to this drug in neonates.
   4. Fat is the only compartment in which thiopental continues to accumulate 30 minutes after injection.
D. **Effects on organ systems**
   1. **Cardiovascular.** Induction doses cause a decrease in blood pressure and an elevation in heart rate. Tachycardia is probably due to a central vagolytic effect.
   2. **Respiratory.** Barbiturate depression on the medullary ventilatory center decreases the ventilatory response to hypercapnia and hypoxia. Laryngospasm and hiccuping are more common after methohexital than after thiopental.
   3. **Cerebral.** Barbiturates constrict cerebral vasculature, decreasing cerebral blood flow and intracranial pressure. Barbiturates cause a decline in cerebral oxygen consumption (up to 50% of normal) and

slowing of the EEG. This effect may provide some brain protection from transient episodes of focal ischemia (eg, cerebral embolism), but probably not from global ischemia (eg, cardiac arrest).
   4. **Renal.** Barbiturates decrease renal blood flow and glomerular filtration rate in proportion to the fall in blood pressure.
   5. **Hepatic.** Hepatic blood flow is decreased.
  E. **Adverse effects**
   1. Barbiturates are contraindicated in patients with acute intermittent porphyria, variegate porphyria, and hereditary coprophyria.
   2. Venous irritation and tissue damage.
   3. Myoclonus and hiccuping.
II. **Ketamine**
  A. **Mechanism of action.** Ketamine blocks polysynaptic reflexes in the spinal cord, inhibiting excitatory neurotransmitter effects. Ketamine functionally dissociates the thalamus from the limbic cortex, producing a state of dissociative anesthesia.
  B. **Structure.** Ketamine is a structural analogue of phencyclidine (PCP).
  C. **Pharmacokinetics.** Metabolized in the liver to multiple metabolites.
  D. **Effects on organ systems**
   1. **Cardiovascular.** Ketamine increases arterial blood pressure, heart rate, and cardiac output. Ketamines direct myocardial depressant effects (large doses) are unmasked by sympathetic blockade or patients who are catecholamine depleted.
   2. **Respiratory.** Ventilation is minimally affected with normal doses of ketamine. Ketamine is a potent bronchodilator.
   3. **Cerebral.** Ketamine increases cerebral oxygen consumption, cerebral blood flow, and intracranial pressure.
  E. **Drug interactions.** Nondepolarizing muscle relaxants are potentiated by ketamine. The combination of ketamine and theophylline may predispose patients to seizures.
  F. **Adverse effects**
   1. Increased salivation (can be attenuated by pretreatment with an anticholinergic).
   2. Delirium. Unpleasant dreams occur for up to 24 hours. These can be reduced by benzodiazepine premedication.
   3. Myoclonic movements.
   4. Increased ICP.
   5. Eyes. nystagmus, diplopia, blepharospasm, and increased intraocular pressure.
III. **Etomidate**
  A. **Mechanisms of action.** Etomidate depresses the reticular activating system and mimics the inhibitory effects of gamma-aminobutyric acid. The disinhibitory effects of etomidate on the parts of the nervous system that control extrapyramidal motor activity contribute to a high incidence of myoclonus.
  B. **Pharmacokinetics.** Like other barbiturates, redistribution is responsible for decreasing the plasma concentration to awakening levels. Biotransformation is five times greater for etomidate than for thiopental.
  C. **Effects on organ systems**
   1. **Cardiovascular.** Minimal cardiovascular changes are seen.
   2. **Respiratory.** Ventilation is less affected with etomidate than

Pharmacology 51

thiopental.
3. **Cerebral.** Decreases the cerebral metabolic rate, cerebral blood flow, and intracranial pressure.
4. **Endocrine.** induction doses of etomidate transiently inhibit enzymes involved in cortisol and aldosterone synthesis. Long term infusions lead to adrenocortical suppression.

D. **Drug interactions.** Fentanyl increases the plasma level and prolongs the elimination half-life of etomidate.

E. **Adverse effects**
1. Myoclonic movements on induction, opioids levels are decreased.
2. High incidence of nausea and vomiting.
3. Venous irritation due to propylene glycol additive.
4. Adrenal suppression.

IV. **Propofol**
A. **Mechanisms of action.** Propofol increases the inhibitory neurotransmission mediated by gamma-aminobutyric acid.
B. **Pharmacokinetics.** Highly lipid solubility. Short duration of action results from a very short initial distribution half-life (2-8 minutes). Elimination occurs primarily through hepatic metabolism to inactive metabolites. Recovery from propofol is more rapid and accompanied by less hangover than other induction agents.
C. **Effects on organ systems**
1. **Cardiovascular.** Decrease in arterial blood pressure secondary to a drop in systemic vascular resistance, contractility, and preload. Hypotension is more pronounced than with thiopental. Propofol markedly impairs the normal arterial baroreflex response to hypotension.
2. **Respiratory.** Propofol causes profound respiratory depression. Propofol induced depression of upper airway reflexes exceeds that of thiopental.
3. **Cerebral.** Decreases cerebral blood flow and intracranial pressure. Propofol has antiemetic and antipruritic properties.

D. **Other effects**
1. Venous irritation. Pain may be reduced by prior administration of opioids or lidocaine.
2. Propofol is an emulsion and should be used with caution if lipid disorder present. Propofol is preservative free.
3. Very low incidence of anaphylaxis; caution with egg allergy.
4. Occasional myoclonic movement.

Inhaled Anesthetics

I. **Ventilation effects of inhalational anesthetics**
A. **Breathing patterns.** Increased respiratory rate (due to CNS stimulation); decreased tidal volume; decreased minute ventilation (increased respiratory rate insufficient to compensate for decrease TV); overall breathing pattern: rapid, shallow, rhythmic, and regular.
B. **PaCO$_2$.** Dose dependent increase except for nitrous (enflurane > halothane or isoflurane); lessens with time.
C. **Ventilatory responsiveness to PaCO$_2$.** Threshold increased, decrease slope, decrease sensitivity to PaCO$_2$ (nitrous has least effect).

52 Pharmacology

D. Ventilatory response to decreasing PaO$_2$. Inhaled anesthetics inhibit hypoxic drive of carotid body.

E. Bronchodilation. Probably due to CNS depression or blocking of afferent nerves.

Inhaled Anesthetics

Agent	MAC[1]	Blood:gas coefficient[2]	Vapor pressure[3]	Metabolism (%)[4]
Methoxyflurane	0.16	12.0	22.5	50
Isoflurane	1.15	1.4	240	0.2
Enflurane	1.68	1.9	172	2-5
Halothane	0.75	2.4	244	15-20
Desflurane	7.25	0.42	669	<0.1
Sevoflurane	2.05	0.68	160	2%
Nitrous Oxide	105-110	0.46		0.0004

1=Minimum alveolar concentration at one atmosphere at which 50% of patients do not move in response to a surgical skin incision.
2=Blood:gas partition coefficient is inversely related to the rate of induction.
3=Vapor pressure is reported as mmHg at 20°C.
4=Percentage of absorbed anesthetic undergoing metabolism.

Circulatory Effects of Inhaled Anesthetics

	Isoflurane/ Desflurane	Halothane	Enflurane	Nitrous Oxide
Cardiac Output	0	-*	-*	+
Heart Rate	++/0	0	++*	*
Blood Pressure	--*	-*	--*	+
Stroke Volume	-*	-*	--*	-
Contractility	--*	---*	--*	-*
System Vascular Resistance	--	0	-	0
Pulmonary Vascular Resistance	0	0	0	+
Coronary Blood Flow	+	0	0	0
Cerebral Blood Flow	+	+++	+	0
Catecholamine Levels	0	0	0	0

*=Dose dependent; -=decrease; --=large decrease; 0=no change; +=increase; ++=large

increase.

II. Circulatory effects of inhalational anesthetics
A. Blood pressure
1. A greater decrease occurs with isoflurane and enflurane than with halothane; no change with nitrous. Desflurane and sevoflurane also decrease blood pressure in dose-dependent fashion.
2. Halothane and enflurane. Decrease contractility and CO.
3. Isoflurane. Decrease SVR and vasodilatation.

B. Heart rate
1. Halothane. No change (baroreceptors inhibited).
2. Isoflurane. Increase by as much as 20% (dose independent increase effect above 1 MAC).
3. Enflurane. Only anesthetic with dose dependent increase (reflex tachycardia via baroreceptor).
4. Nitrous Oxide. Minimally increased.
5. Desflurane and sevoflurane. Increased.

C. Cardiac output.
Halothane, but not the other inhalational anesthetics, decreases cardiac output in a dose dependent fashion. No change to slight increase with nitrous oxide.

D. Stroke volume.
All inhaled anesthetics cause a dose dependent reduction (greatest with enflurane), except nitrous (no change).

E. Contractility.
Decrease with halothane and enflurane (minimal change with isoflurane).

F. Systemic vascular resistance.
Decrease with isoflurane, desflurane, sevoflurane and enflurane; no change with nitrous or halothane.

G. Pulmonary vascular resistance.
Nitrous increases PVR (especially in patients with pulmonary HTN); halothane, enflurane, and isoflurane have minimal effect.

H. Right atrial pressure.
Increase with nitrous (due to increase in PVR), enflurane and halothane; minimal to no change with isoflurane due to its peripheral vasodilating effects.

I. Coronary resistance.
Decrease with isoflurane (coronary steal syndrome), no significant change with halothane or enflurane, autoregulation remains intact.

J. Cardiac dysrhythmias.
Most with halothane and least with enflurane; halothane, enflurane, and isoflurane all slow conduction through the A-V node; halothane slows conduction through His-Purkinje fibers and is not dose related (arrhythmias should not be treated by decreasing halothane).

III. Metabolic effects of inhalational anesthetics
A. Halothane.
Primarily metabolism (mainly oxidative) and ventilation; oxidative metabolism results in trifluroacetic acid and bromide (Br concentration increases 0.5 mEq/L/MAC hr) with CNS toxicity (somnolence, confusion) occurring with levels greater then 6.0 mEqL; reductive metabolism (occurs with hypoxia or induction of microsomal enzymes) results in reactive intermediates and fluoride.

B. Enflurane.
Primarily ventilation; minimal metabolism (reduction); oxidative metabolism results in fluoride; enzyme induction with phenobarbital does not increase defluoridation; defluoridation is increased in patients on chronic INH therapy.

C. Isoflurane.
Primarily ventilation; oxidative metabolism results in trifluroacetic acid and difluromethanol (which is unstable, leading to

formic acid and fluoride); enzyme induction does not significantly increase metabolism.

D. Methoxyflurane. Primarily metabolism (oxidation); major metabolite is fluoride; serum fluoride concentration is lower in pediatric patients due to bone uptake.

E. Nitrous oxide. Primarily ventilation; minimal reductive metabolism in GI tract by anaerobic bacteria (pseudomonas).

F. Desflurane. Primarily ventilation; no evidence of nephrotoxic effects. Metabolism of inhalational anesthetics is dependent on the cytochrome P-450 enzyme, which can by induced by drugs. Obesity is associated with increased defluoridation.

IV. Fluoride induced nephrotoxicity

A. Nephrotoxicity is seen with fluoride levels greater then 50 uM/L (toxic levels of fluoride may be seen after 2.5 MAC hrs of methoxyflurane or 9.6 MAC hrs of enflurane). Fluoride nephrotoxicity depends on the duration of exposure of renal tubules to fluoride and the absolute level.

B. Fluoride elimination is dependent on GFR. Fluoride nephrotoxicity may result in inability to concentrate urine.

V. Inhaled anesthetics. miscellaneous information

A. Nitrous oxide is colorless; odorless; good analgesic.

B. Halothane is colorless, poor analgesic; bronchodilation; hypotension (secondary to peripheral vasodilation, myocardial depression; sympathetic ganglionic blockade; and inhibition of the baroreceptor reflex); can cause uterine relaxation; preferentially depresses intercostal muscles more than diaphragm.

C. Enflurane has a pleasant odor; slightly irritating to upper airways; 2% of patients exhibit EEG patterns of seizure activity.

D. Isoflurane is the least blood soluble agent and is the least potent cardiac depressant; good for controlled hypotension; least increase in cerebral blood flow.

E. Desflurane is similar in structure to isoflurane. It has an ultrashort duration of action and moderate potency.

Drugs and Drips

Adenosine (Adenocard)

Actions. Adenosine slows conduction through the A-V node.

Indications. Paroxysmal supraventricular tachycardia, Wolf-Parkinson-White syndrome

Dose. 6 mg rapid IV bolus; may be repeated within 1-2 minutes with 12 mg (up to two doses). Children 0.05-0.25 mg/kg.

Adverse effects. The effects are antagonized by methylxanthines.

Misc. Contraindicated in patients with second or third-degree heart block or sick sinus syndrome. Large doses given by infusion may cause hypotension. Not effective in atrial flutter or fibrillation.

Aminocaproic Acid (Amicar)

Actions. Inhibits plasminogen activators (fibrinolysis inhibitor).

Indications. Excessive acute bleeding from hyperfibrinolysis, chronic bleeding tendency; antidote for excessive thrombolysis.

Dose. Loading dose of 100-150 mg/kg IV over the first 30-60 minutes followed by constant infusion of 1 gm/hour for about 8 hours or until bleeding controlled. Most common regimen for adult: 5 gram loading (started prior to skin incision) followed by constant infusion of 1 gm/hour.

Adverse effects. Contraindicated in patients with active intravascular clotting, DIC, and bleeding in the kidneys or ureters; hypotension, bradycardia, dysrhythmias, elevated LFT's, thrombosis.

Aminophylline

Actions. Inhibits of phosphodiesterase, resulting in bronchodilation with positive inotropic and chronotropic effects.

Loading dose. 5-7 mg/kg IVPB over 15-30 min (6 mg/kg PO).

Maintenance (IV).
1) Children 1-9 years 1 mg/kg/hr
2) Children >9 years 0.8 mg/kg/hr
3) Adult smokers 0.8 mg/kg/hr
4) Adult non-smokers 0.5 mg/kg/hr
5) Adults w/CHF/liver 0.25 mg/kg/hr

Rate determination. cc/hr = dose x body wt (kg) when mixed 1 mg/kg.

Therapeutic level. 10-20 mg/dL.

Adverse effects. Nausea, vomiting, anorexia, dizziness, headaches, agitation, tachyarrhythmias, ventricular arrhythmias, palpitations, overdosage hyperreflexia, convulsions, hypotension, tachypnea.

Misc. Aminophylline contains about 80% theophylline by weight.

Amiodarone (Cordarone)

Actions. Depresses the sinoatrial node, prolongs the PR, QRS, and QT intervals, and produces alpha- and beta-adrenergic blockade.

Indications. Refractory or recurrent ventricular tachycardia or VF.

Dosage. Loading dose of 800-1600 mg/day PO x 1-3 weeks, then 600-800 mg/day PO x 4 weeks.

Adverse effects. May cause severe sinus bradycardia, ventricular dysrhythmias, AV block, liver and thyroid function test abnormalities, hepatitis, and cirrhosis. Pulmonary fibrosis may follow long-term use. Increases serum levels of digoxin, oral anticoagulants, diltiazem, quinidine, procainamide, and phenytoin.

Amrinone (Inocor)

Actions. Phosphodiesterase inhibitor (rapid inotropic agent) causing increase in cardiac output while pulmonary vascular resistance and preload decrease (positive inotropic and vasodilator properties).

Indications. Severe CHF not responding to conventional therapy.

Dosage. Loading dose of 0.75 mg/kg is given over 3-5 minutes, followed by a 2-20 mcg/kg/min infusion.

Standard conc. 100 mg in 250 cc NS (do not mix in dextrose solutions).

Adverse effects. Worsening myocardial ischemia, thrombocytopenia; contraindicated if allergic to bisulfites; hepatic function abnormalities, nausea, vomiting, hypotension, arrhythmias.

Misc. Do not dilute in dextrose containing solutions; do not administer furosemide (Lasix) in same IV line.

Aprotinin (Trasylol)

Actions. Inhibitor of several proteases (including trypsin, kallikrein, and plasmin) and inhibits factor XIIa activation of complement.

Indications. Prophylactic use to reduce bleeding and transfusion requirements in high-risk cardiac surgery patients.

Test dose. 1 mL (1.4 mg) administer IV at least 10 minutes before loading dose. After the test dose is given, either the low dose regimen (100 cc load followed by 25 cc/hr maintenance) or high dose (200 cc load followed by 50 cc/hr maintenance) regimen may be started.

Loading dose. 100 cc (140 mg) or 200 mL (280 mg) IV, slowly over 20-30 minutes with patient in supine position.

Maintenance. 25 (35 mg/hr) or 50 mL/hr (70 mg/hr) started after loading dose is completed.

Adverse effects. Allergic reactions and anaphylaxis.

Misc. Aprotinin prolongs whole blood clotting time of heparinized blood (prolonged PTT). Patients may require additional heparin even in the presence of activated clotting time (ACT) levels that appear to represent adequate anticoagulation. All doses of aprotinin should be administered through a central line. No other drugs should be administer in the same line.

Atropine

Actions. Competitive blockade of acetylcholine at muscarinic receptors.
Indications. bradycardia and antisialagogue.
Dose. Antisialagogue: adult 0.2-0.4 mg IV; pediatric 0.01 mg/kg/dose IV/IM
Bradycardia. adult 0.4 mg IV; pediatric 0.02 mg/kg IV.
Adverse effects. May cause tachydysrhythmias, AV dissociation, premature ventricular contractions, dry mouth, or urinary retention. CNS effects occur at high doses.

Bicarbonate (Sodium Bicarbonate)

Actions. Hydrogen ion neutralization.
Indications. metabolic acidosis.
Dose. IV dose in mEq $NaHCO_3$ = [base deficit x weight (kg) x 0.3]
Adverse effects. May cause metabolic alkalosis, hypercarbia, hyperosmolality. May decrease cardiac output, systemic vascular resistance, and myocardial contractility. Crosses placenta. 8.4% solution is approximately 1.0 mEq/mL. 4.2% solution is approximately 0.5 mEq/mL.

Bretylium (Bretylol)

Actions. Initially, release of norepinephrine into circulation, followed by prevention of synaptic release of norepinephrine; suppression of ventricular fibrillation and ventricular arrhythmias; increase in myocardial contractility (direct effect).
Indications. Ventricular fibrillation and ventricular tachycardia.
Dose. 5 mg/kg IV push initially, followed by 5-10 mg/kg every 15-30 min to total of 30 mg/kg.
Continuous infusion. 1-2 mg/min (2 gm/500 cc D_5W at 30 cc/hr).
Adverse effects. Postural hypotension (potentiated by quinidine or procainamide), aggravation of digoxin induced arrhythmias, nausea/vomiting following rapid injection.

Bumetanide (Bumex)

Actions. Loop diuretic with principal effect on the ascending limb of the loop of Henle. Causes increased excretion of Na, K, and Cl, and H_2O.
Indications. Edema, hypertension, intracranial hypertension.
Dose. 0.5-1.0 mg IV, repeated to a maximum of 10 mg/day.

Adverse effects. May cause electrolyte imbalance, dehydration, and deafness. Patients who are allergic to sulfonamides may show hypersensitivity to bumetanide. Effective in renal insufficiency.

Calcium
Actions. Essential for maintenance of cell membrane integrity, muscular excitation-contraction coupling, glandular stimulation-secretion coupling, and enzyme function.
Indications. Hypocalcemia, hyperkalemia, hypomagnesemia, hypotension.
Dose. 500-1000 mg calcium chloride (2-10 mg/kg IV); 10% $CaCl_2$=1.36 mEq Ca^2/mL.
Adverse effects. May cause bradycardia or arrhythmia (especially with digitalis), hypertension, increased risk of ventricular fibrillation, and can be irritating to veins.

Citrate (Bicitra)
Actions. Absorbed and metabolized to sodium bicarbonate.
Indications. Gastric acid neutralization.
Dose. 15-60 cc PO
Adverse effects. Contraindicated in patients with sodium restriction or severe renal impairment. Do not use with aluminum based antacids.

Dantrolene (Dantrium)
Actions. Reduction of calcium release from sarcoplasmic reticulum.
Indications. Malignant hyperthermia, skeletal muscle spasticity.
Dose. 3 mg/kg IV bolus; if syndrome persists after 30 minutes, repeat dose, up to 10 mg/kg (see section on malignant hyperthermia).
Adverse effects. Muscle weakness, gastrointestinal upset, drowsiness, sedation, or abnormal liver function. Additive effect with neuromuscular blocking agents.
Comments. Mix 20 mg in 60 cc of sterile water. Dissolves slowly.

Desmopressin Acetate (DDAVP)
Actions. Synthetic product that increases plasma levels of Factor VIII and von Willebrand factor (vWF) and decreases bleeding times; causes release of tissue plasminogen activator and prostacyclin; antidiuretic activity.
Indications. Bleeding uremic patients with platelet dysfunction, cirrhosis, cardiac surgery; improves coagulation in von Willebrand's disease and hemophilia; used as a antidiuretic hormone.
Dose. 0.3 mcg/kg IV over 20 minutes.
Adverse effects. Decreased free water clearance from antidiuretic activity, hypotension, thrombosis, decreased serum sodium.

Dexamethasone (Decadron)
Actions. Antiinflammatory and antiallergic effects. Has 25 times the glucocorticoid potency of hydrocortisone.
Indications. Cerebral edema from CNS tumors; airway edema.
Dose. Load 10 mg IV; maintenance 4 mg IV q6 hours.
Adverse effects. May cause adrenocortical insufficiency (Addison's crisis) with abrupt withdrawal, delayed wound healing, CNS disturbances, osteoporosis, and electrolyte disturbances.

58 Pharmacology

Dextran 40 (Rheomacrodex)
Actions. Immediate, short-lived plasma volume expansion; prevents RBC aggregation, decreasing blood viscosity and platelet adhesiveness.
Indications. Inhibition of platelet aggregation; improvement of blood flow in low-flow states (eg, vascular surgery); intravascular volume expander.
Dose. Adult: load 30-50 mL IV over 30 min, maintenance 15-30 mL/hr; pediatric: <20 mL/kg/24 hr of 10% dextran.
Adverse effects. May cause volume overload, anaphylaxis, bleeding tendency, interference with blood cross matching, or false elevation of blood glucose level. Can cause renal failure.

Digoxin
Actions. (1) positive inotropic effects; (2) negative chronotropic effects; (3) slows conduction velocity through the AV node.
Pharmacokinetics. Onset of action is about 30 min following IV.
Indications. CHF, heart rate control in atrial fib/flutter.
Dose. (1) for supraventricular tachycardia: 10-15 mcg/kg IV in divided doses (0.25-0.5 mg as initial dose and 0.25 mg every 4 hours as subsequent doses until the entire dose is given or heart rate controlled); (2) CHF: 8-12 mcg/kg given in divided doses as above.
Therapeutic level. 0.8-2.0 ng/mL.
Adverse effects. Symptoms of digoxin toxicity include mental depression, confusion, headaches, drowsiness, anorexia, nausea, vomiting, weakness, visual disturbances, delirium, EKG abnormalities (any arrhythmia) and seizures. Hypokalemia increases risk of digoxin toxicity. Heart block potentiated by beta blockers or calcium channel blockers.

Diltiazem (Cardizem)
Actions. Calcium channel antagonist; slows conduction through sinoatrial and AV nodes; dilates coronary and peripheral arterioles, and reduces myocardial contractility.
Indications. Angina pectoris, temporary control of rapid ventricular rate during atrial fibrillation/flutter; conversion of paroxysmal supraventricular tachycardia to normal sinus rhythm.
Dose. (1) PO: 30-60 mg every 6 hours; (2) IV: initial bolus with 0.25 mg/kg over 2 minutes; if response is inadequate after 15 minutes, rebolus with 0.35 mg/kg over 2 minutes; for treatment give continuous infusion 5-15 mg/h (mix 125 mg in 100 cc of D_5W).
Adverse effects. Bradycardia and heart block; impaired contractility; transient increase in liver function tests. Adverse events include hypotension, injection site reaction, flushing, and arrhythmia. Contraindicated in atrial fib/flutter patients with WPW or short PR syndrome; sick sinus syndrome or second- or third-degree AV block except with a pacemaker.

Diphenhydramine (Benadryl)
Actions. Antagonism of histamine action on H_1 receptors; anticholinergic; CNS depression.
Indications. Allergenic reactions, extrapyramidal reactions, sedation.
Dose. adult: 10-50 mg IV q6-8 hours; pediatric: 5.0 mg/kg/day IV in four divided doses (maximum of 300 mg).
Adverse effects. May cause hypotension, tachycardia, dizziness, urinary retention, seizures.

Dobutamine (Dobutrex)
Action. Beta 1 and beta 2 adrenergic agonist (greater increase in myocardial contractility than increase in heart rate); alpha-1-adrenergic agonist (beta 2 effect greater than alpha 1 effect; decreases systemic and pulmonary vascular resistance).
Indications. Cardiogenic shock, severe CHF; low cardiac output.
Standard concentration. 250 mg/250 D5W (1 mg/cc).
Dose. 2-20 mcg/kg/min. Drip rate: 15 cc/hr = 250 mcg/min.
Adverse effects. Tachycardia (less than dopamine); minimal ventricular ectopy; hypertension. Can increase ventricular rate in atrial fibrillation.

Dolasetron Mesylate (Anzemet)
Actions. Serotonin receptor antagonist.
Indications. Postoperative nausea and vomiting.
Dose. 12.5 mg IV; 100 mg PO.
Adverse effects. May cause headaches, dizziness, and hypertension. Use with caution in patients who have or may develop prolongation of cardiac conduction intervals, particularly QTc.

Dopamine (Intropin)
Actions. Dopaminergic, alpha and beta adrenergic agonist
Indications. Shock, poor perfusion, decreased splanchnic perfusion, low cardiac output.
Standard conc. 400 mg/250 cc D5W = 1600 mcg/cc.
Dosage range. 2-20 mcg/kg/min
  2-5 mcg/kg/min: dopamine, minimal beta 1 stimulation B1
  5-10 mcg/kg/min: B1 > alpha
  10-15 mcg/kg/min: alpha > B1
  >15 mcg/kg/min: alpha agonist
Drip rate. 15 cc/hr = 400 mcg/min
Adverse effects. Tachycardia, arrhythmias, nausea/vomiting; superficial tissue necrosis and sloughing may occur with extravasation, contraindicated in pheochromocytoma

Dopexamine
Actions. Synthetic analogue of dopamine, beta-2 and dopamine agonist (little beta-1 or alpha activity).
Indications. Shock, poor perfusion, decreased splanchnic perfusion, low cardiac output, oliguria.
Dose. 1-10 mcg/kg/min.
Adverse effects. Hypotension (causes vasodilation), tachycardia (atrial).

Droperidol
Actions. Dopamine (D_2) receptor antagonist, antiemetic effect, antipsychotic effect, apparent psychic indifference to environment.
Indications. Nausea, vomiting, agitation, sedation
Dose (adult) antiemetic. 0.625-2.5 mg prn; sedation: 2.5-10 mg IV prn.
Dose (pediatric) antiemetic. 0.05-0.06 mg/kg q4-6 hours.
Adverse effects. Evokes extrapyramidal reactions in 1%; possible dysphoric reactions; cerebral vasoconstrictor; can decrease blood pressure by alpha blockade and dopaminergic antagonism, used in neuroleptanalgesia, potentiates other CNS depressants.

60 Pharmacology

Ephedrine
Actions. Alpha- and beta-adrenergic stimulation; norepinephrine release at sympathetic nerve endings (indirect).
Indications. Hypotension.
Dose. 5-50 mg IV prn
Adverse effects. May cause hypertension, dysrhythmias, myocardial ischemia. Avoid giving to patients taking monoamine oxidase inhibitors. Tachyphylaxis with repeated dosing.

Epinephrine (Adrenalin)
Actions. Direct alpha and beta adrenergic receptor stimulation, resulting in bronchial smooth muscle relaxation and cardiac stimulation (positive inotrope).
Indications. Heart failure, hypotension, cardiac arrest, bronchospasm, anaphylaxis.
Standard conc. 2 mg/250 cc (15 cc/hr = 2 mcg/min).
Dose (cardiac arrest, hypotension). 0.1-1 mg IV or intracardiac q5 minute prn; 1 mg intratracheal prn.
Dose (bronchospasm). 0.1-0.5 mg SQ q10-15 min or 0.1-0.25 mg IV.
Dose (infusion). Start at 2 mcg/min (or 0.05 mcg/kg/min) and titrate to blood pressure and cardiac output; bolus starting at 10-20 mcg; infusion 0.01- 0.3 mcg/kg/min.
Dose (pediatric-neonates). 0.01-0.3 mg/kg q3-5 minutes.
Dose (children). 0.01 mg/kg IV or intratracheal q3-5 minutes; 0.01 mg/kg SQ q15 minutes for bronchospasm.
Adverse effects. May cause hypertension, dysrhythmias, or myocardial ischemia. Dysrhythmias potentiated by halothane. Crosses placenta.

Epinephrine, racemic (Vaponefrin)
Actions. Mucosal vasoconstriction (see epinephrine).
Indications. Airway edema, bronchospasm.
Dose. Inhaled via nebulizer: 0.5 mL of 2.25% solution in 2.5-3.5 mL of NSS q1-4 hr prn.
Adverse effects. See epinephrine.

Ergonovine (Ergotrate)
Actions. Constriction of uterine and vascular smooth muscle.
Indications. Postpartum uterine atony and bleeding, uterine involution.
Dose. 0.2 mg IV in 5 mL NS given over 1 minute (IV route is used only in emergencies). 0.2 mg IM q2-4 hours for less than 5 doses; then PO: O.2-0.4 mg q6-12 hours for 2 days.
Adverse effects. May cause hypertension from system vasoconstriction, arrhythmias, coronary spasm, cerebrovascular accidents, uterine tetany, or gastrointestinal upset.

Esmolol (Brevibloc)
Actions. Short acting selective beta-1 adrenergic blockade.
Indications. Supraventricular tachyarrhythmias, myocardial ischemia.
Dose (bolus). 5-100 mg IV prn.
Dose (infusion). Load 500 mcg/kg bolus over 1 min followed by maintenance starting at 50 mcg/kg/min (1-15 mg/min). To calculate an infusion rate in mL/min, divide mg/min by 10. To calculate an infusion rate in mL/hr,

multiply mg/min by 6.
Standard conc. 10 mg/mL (infusion mix two 2.5 gm ampuls in 500 cc).
Adverse effects. Bradycardia, AV conduction delay, hypotension, congestive heart failure.

Etomidate (Amidate)

Actions. Augments the inhibitory tone of GABA in the CNS (produces unconsciousness in approximately 30 seconds).
Indications. IV induction agent for general anesthesia.
Induction. 0.2-0.3 mg/kg IV.
Maintenance. 10 mcg/kg/min IV with N 20 and opiate.
Sedation and analgesia. 5-8 mcg/kg/min; used only for short periods of time due to inhibition of corticosteroid synthesis.
Adverse effects. Direct cerebral vasoconstrictor, minimal cardiovascular effects, pain on injection, myoclonus may occur in about 1/3 of patients during induction, adrenocortical suppression, nausea/vomiting.

Flumazenil (Romazicon)

Actions. Competitive inhibition of GABA.
Indications. Reversal of benzodiazepine sedation or overdose.
Dose. (1) for reversal of conscious sedation: 0.2-1.0 mg IV every 20 minutes at 0.2 mg/min, (2) for overdose: 3-5 mg IV at 0.5 mg/min.
Adverse effects. Seizures, acute withdrawal, nausea, dizziness, agitation, arrhythmias, hypertension.
Drug interactions. Seizures in patients with prior seizure activity, tricyclic antidepressant poisoning, major hypnotic drug withdrawal.

Furosemide (Lasix)

Actions. Increase in excretion of sodium and potassium and water by inhibiting reabsorption in the loop of Henle.
Indications. Edema, hypertension, intracranial hypertension, renal failure, hypercalcemia.
Dose (adult). 2-100 mg IV; pediatric: 1-2 mg/kg/day.
Adverse effects. May cause electrolyte imbalance, dehydration, transient hypotension, deafness, hyperglycemia, or hyperuricemia.

Heparin

Actions. Heparin, prepared from bovine lung, facilitates the activation of anti-thrombin III, neutralizes primarily thrombin and factor X.
Indications. Anticoagulation.
Loading dose. (1) for thromboembolism: 5000 units IVP, (2) for cardiopulmonary bypass: 300 units/kg.
Maintenance dose. (1) for thromboembolism: start 1000 units/hr and titrate to PTT 1.5 to 2.5 x control, (2) for cardiopulmonary bypass: 100 units/kg/hr IV titrated against activated clotting time.
Standard conc. 10,000 units/500 cc D_5W (20 units per cc).
Reversal. Reverse with protamine sulfate.
Adverse effects. Hemorrhage, allergic reactions, thrombocytopenia, altered protein binding, decreased MAP, decreased antithrombin III concentration, altered cell morphology, does not cross placenta.

Hydralazine (Apresoline)
Actions. Relaxation of vascular smooth muscle.
Indications. Hypertension.
Dose. 2.5-20 mg IV q4 hr or prn.
Adverse effects. Hypotension, reflex tachycardia, systemic lupus erythematosus syndrome, or Coombs' test positive hemolytic anemia.

Hydrocortisone (SoluCortef)
Actions. Anti-inflammatory and antiallergic effects. Mineralocorticoid effect. Stimulation of gluconeogenesis. Inhibition of peripheral protein synthesis.
Indications. Adrenal insufficiency, inflammation and allergy, cerebral edema from CNS tumors, asthma.
Dose. Non-life threatening conditions: 50-200 mg IV q2-10 hrs prn. Life threatening conditions: 50 mg/kg IV over several minutes q4-24 hrs.
Adverse effects. May cause adrenocortical insufficiency (Addison's crisis) with abrupt withdrawal, delayed wound healing, CNS disturbances, osteoporosis, or electrolyte disturbances.

Indigo Carmine (Indigotindisulfonate Sodium)
Actions. Rapid glomerular filtration causing blue urine.
Indications. Evaluation of urine output. Localizing of ureteral orifices during surgery.
Dose. 40 mg IV slowly (5 mL of 0.8% solution).
Adverse effects. Hypertension from alpha adrenergic stimulation, lasts 15-30 minutes after IV dose.

Insulin
Indications. Hyperglycemia.
Actions. Facilitation of glucose transport into cells.
Infusion. 50 units regular insulin in 250 cc D_5W or NS (1 U/hr = 5 cc/hr).
Dose. Average range is 2-10 units/hour or 0.1 units/kg/hour.
Adverse effects. Hypoglycemia, allergic reactions, absorbed by IV tubing.

Isoproterenol (Isuprel)
Actions. Synthetic sympathomimetic amine that acts on beta-1 and beta-2 adrenergic receptors; positive chronotrope and inotrope; decreases systemic and pulmonary vascular resistance; increases coronary and renal blood flow.
Indications. Bradycardia, shock where increasing HR will increase CO, shock with severe aortic regurgitation, heart failure, pulmonary hypertension, refractory asthma, carotid sinus hypersensitivity.
Dose. 2-20 mcg/min; start at 1-2 mcg/min; peds: 0.01 mcg/kg/min.
Standard conc. 1 mg/250 cc; 15 cc = 1 mcg.
Adverse effects. Arrhythmogenic, especially with cardiac ischemia and digoxin toxicity; hypertension, CNS excitation, nausea/vomiting; pulmonary edema; paradoxical precipitation of Adams-Stokes attacks.

Ketamine
Induction
0.5-2 mg/kg IV; 4-6 mg/kg IM
Maintenance
0.5-1 mg/kg IV prn with nitrons 20 50%
15-45 mcg/kg/min IV with nitrons 20 50-70%

30-90 mcg/kg/min IV without nitrons 20
 Sedation and analgesia
 0.2-0.8 mg/kg IV; 2-4 mg/kg IM; 3 mg/kg intranasally; 6-10 mg/kg PO
 Adverse effects. Causes increased HR, CO, cardiac work, and myocardial oxygen requirements; direct stimulation of the CNS leads to increased sympathetic nervous system outflow. Ketamine is a direct myocardial depressant, potent cerebral vasodilator, and it should not be used in patients receiving aminophylline (reduces seizure threshold).

Ketorolac (Toradol)

Action. Inhibits prostaglandin synthesis through cyclo-oxygenase inhibition.
Indications: nonopioid, nonsteroidal analgesic for moderate pain.

Single dose (IM). Patients <65 years of age: 60 mg; patients >65 years of age, renally impaired and/or less than 50 kg: 30 mg.

Single dose (IV). Patients <65 years of age: one dose of 30 mg; patients >65 years of age, renally impaired and/or less than 50 kg: one dose of 15 mg.

Multiple dosing (IV or IM). Patients <65 years of age: 30 mg every 6 hours. The maximum daily dose should not exceed 120 mg. For patients >65 years of age, renally impaired and patients less than 50 kg should have one-half the above dose. The combined duration of use for parenteral and oral should not exceed 5 days.

Adverse effects. Adverse effects are similar to those of other nonsteroidal anti-inflammatory drugs and include peptic ulceration. Contraindicated in patients with active peptic ulcer disease, and renal impairment.

Labetalol (Normodyne, Trandate)

Action. Selective alpha-1-adrenergic blockade with nonselective beta-adrenergic blockade

Indications. Hypertension, angina, controlled hypotension.

Dose. 5-10 mg increments at 5 min intervals, to 40-80 mg/dose.

Adverse effects. May cause bradycardia, AV conduction delay, bronchospasm in asthmatics, and postural hypotension.

Lidocaine

Action. Antiarrhythmic effect; sedation; neural blockade.

Loading dose. 1-1.5 mg/kg IVP.

Maintenance. Infusion 1-4 mg/min (reduce by half for patients with CHF, hepatic dysfunction, or shock).

Standard concentration. 2 gm/250 cc; (7 cc/hr = 1 mg/min).

Adverse effects. CNS depression, drowsiness, unconsciousness, apprehension, change in vision, vomiting, bradycardia, hypotension, respiratory depression. Avoid in patients with Wolff-Parkinson-White syndrome.

Magnesium

Actions. Central nervous system depressant and anticonvulsant, inhibits release of acetylcholine at the neuromuscular junction, decreases sensitivity of motor end-plate to acetylcholine, decreases muscle excitability, decreases uterine hyperactivity (thus increasing uterine blood flow).

Indications. Pregnancy induced hypertension, hypomagnesemia.

Dose. (1) for treatment of hypomagnesemia: 4-8 gm/100 cc NS or D_5W given over 8 hours; (2) for pregnancy induced hypertension patients: initial

bolus of 2-4 gm in a 20% solution IV over 5 minutes followed by a continuous infusion of 1-2.5 gm/hr (10-20 gm in 1000 cc of D_5W).
Levels. Normal plasma level is 1.5 to 2.2 mEq/l. In the treatment of pregnancy induced hypertension the therapeutic level is 4-5 mEq/l.
Adverse effects. (1) at 5-10 mEq/l: there is loss of deep tendon reflexes and respiratory depression; (2) at 10 mEq/l: there are prolonged PR and QT intervals and widened QRS complexes; (3) at 15 mEq/l: there is SA and AV nodal blocks and respiratory apnea; (4) at 25 mEq/l: cardiac arrest.

Mannitol (Osmitrol)

Actions. Increase in serum osmolality resulting in decrease in brain swelling, osmotic diuresis, and transient expansion of intravascular volume.
Indications. Intracranial hypertension, treatment of renal failure, glaucoma, diuresis.
Dose (adult). 0.25-1.0 gm/kg IV as 20% solution over 30-60 minutes (in acute situation, can give bolus of 1.25-25 gm over 5-10 minutes).
Dose (pediatric). 0.2 g/kg test dose, with maintenance of 2 g/kg over 30-60 minutes.
Adverse effects. Rapid administration may cause vasodilation and hypotension. May cause pulmonary edema, intracranial hemorrhage, systemic hypertension.

Methohexital (Brevital)

Indications. IV induction agent for general anesthesia.
Induction. 1-1.5 mg/kg IV or 20-30 mg/kg pr (children).
Sedation. 0.2-0.4 mg/kg IV.
Adverse effects. Earlier recovery time and less cumulative effect than thiopental, higher incidence of excitatory phenomena (cough, hiccups, involuntary movements), pain on injection, activates epileptic foci (unlike other barbiturates).

Methylene Blue (Urolene Blue)

Actions. Low dose promotes conversion of methemoglobin to hemoglobin. High dose promotes conversion of hemoglobin to methemoglobin. Less useful than sodium nitrate and amyl nitrite.
Indications. Surgical marker for genitourinary surgery, methemoglobinemia.
Dose. Marker: 100 mg (10 mL of 1% solution) IV; methemoglobinemia: 1-2 mg/kg IV. Repeat q1 hr prn.
Adverse effects. May cause RBC destruction (with prolonged use), hypertension, bladder irritation, nausea, diaphoresis. May inhibit nitrate induced coronary artery relaxation. Interferes with pulse oximetry for 1-2 minutes. May cause hemolysis in patients with glucose-6-phosphate-dehydrogenase deficiency.

Methylergonovine (Methergine)

Actions. Constriction of uterine and vascular smooth muscle.
Indications. Postpartum hemorrhage.
Dose. 0.2 mg IV in 5 mL NS given over 1 minute (IV route is used only in emergencies). 0.2 mg IM q2-4 hours for less than 5 doses; then PO: 0.2-0.4 mg q6-12 hours for 2 days.
Adverse effects. May cause hypertension from system vasoconstriction, arrhythmias, coronary spasm, uterine tetany, or gastrointestinal upset.

Methylprednisolone (Solu-Medrol)
Actions. Has 5 times the glucocorticoid potency of hydrocortisone.
Indications. Same as hydrocortisone.
Dose (adult). For non-life threatening conditions: 10-250 mg IV q4-24 hr IV over 1 minute. For life threatening conditions: 100-250 mg IV q2-6 hr or 30 mg/kg IV q4-6 hrs.
Dose (pediatric). For life threatening conditions not <0.5 mg/kg/24 hr.
Adverse effects. See hydrocortisone.

Metoprolol (Lopressor)
Actions. Beta-1 adrenergic blockade (beta-2 adrenergic antagonism at high doses).
Indications. Hypertension, angina pectoris, dysrhythmia, hypertrophic cardiomyopathy, myocardial infarction, pheochromocytoma.
Dose. 50-100 mg PO q4-24 hr.
Adverse effects. May cause bradycardia, clinically significant bronchoconstriction, dizziness, fatigue, insomnia. May increase risk of heart block.

Milrinone (Primacor)
Actions. Phosphodiesterase inhibitor, increases cAMP in the heart, peripheral vasodilator, increases inotropy.
Indications. Low output heart failure.
Loading dose. 50 mcg/kg IV over 10 minutes.
Maintenance dose. 0.375-0.75 mcg/kg/min.
Standard concen. 200 mcg/cc (50 mg/250 cc dextrose or saline).
Adverse effects. Increased ventricular ectopy, nonsustained ventricular tachycardia, supraventricular tachycardia; hypotension; headaches.
Misc. The presence of renal impairment may significantly increase the terminal elimination half-life. Do not inject furosemide into IV lines containing milrinone; a precipitate-forming chemical reaction will occur.

Naloxone (Narcan)
Actions. Antagonism of narcotic effect.
Indications. Reversal of systemic narcotic effects.
Dose (adult). 0.04-0.4 mg IV titrated against patient response q2-3 minutes.
Dose (pediatric). 1-10 mcg/kg q2-3 minutes up to 0.4 mg.
Dose (infusion). 5-10 mcg/kg/hr
Onset/duration. Onset 1-2 minutes; duration less than one hour.
Adverse effects. May cause reversal of analgesia, hypertension, arrhythmias, rare pulmonary edema, delirium or withdrawal syndrome. Renarcotization may occur because of short duration of action.

Nicardipine (Cardene)
Actions. Dihydropyridine calcium channel blocker.
Indications. Short-term treatment of hypertension.
Dose. Administer by slow continuous infusion. Initiate therapy at 50 cc/hr (5.0 mg/hr). If desired blood pressure reduction is not achieved at this dose, the infusion rate may be increased by 25 cc/hr every 5 minutes for rapid blood pressure reduction or every 15 minutes for gradual blood pressure reduction up to a maximum of 150 cc/hr. Following achievement of the blood pressure goal, the infusion rate should be decreased to 30 cc/hr.

66 Pharmacology

Contraindications. Known hypersensitivity to the drug and those with advanced aortic stenosis. Caution when administering in patients with impaired renal or hepatic function or in combination with a beta blocker in CHF patients.

Adverse effects. Most commonly hypotension, headache, tachycardia.

Nifedipine (Procardia)

Actions. Blockade of slow calcium channels in the heart. Systemic and coronary vasodilation and increase in myocardial perfusion.

Indications. Coronary artery spasm, hypertension, myocardial ischemia.

Dose. 10-40 mg PO tid; 10-20 mg SL.

Adverse effects. May cause reflex tachycardia, gastrointestinal tract upset, mild negative inotropic effects. Little effect on automaticity and atrial conduction. Sensitive to light.

Nitroglycerin

Actions. Smooth muscle relaxant; greater venous dilation than arterial dilation (decrease of preload > decrease of afterload), coronary artery dilation, decreased systemic vascular resistance, decreased pulmonary vascular resistance.

Indications. Myocardial ischemia, hypertension, congestive heart failure, pulmonary hypertension, esophageal spasm.

Dose. Start at 5-10 mcg/min and titrate and advance every 5 minutes until chest pain resolved or hemodynamic state achieved.

Standard conc. 50 mg/250 cc; 3 cc/hr = 10 mcg/min.

Adverse effects. Reflex tachycardia, hypotension, headache. Tolerance and dependence with chronic use. May be absorbed by plastic in IV tubing.

Nitroprusside

Actions. Smooth muscle relaxation; arterial dilation greater than venous.

Indications. Hypertension, congestive heart failure, pulmonary hypertension.

Dose. 0.5-10 mcg/kg/min; start at 20 mcg/min. Mix 50 mg/250 cc D_5W.

Adverse effects. Hypotension, nausea, headaches, restlessness, cyanide and thiocyanate toxicity, degraded by light (tubing/container must be covered with aluminum foil), signs of toxicity include tachyphylaxis, metabolic acidosis, and high mixed venous saturation (treatment is with sodium nitrite, sodium thiosulfate, hydroxocobalamin or methylene blue).

Norepinephrine (Levophed)

Actions. Alpha 1, alpha 2, and beta 1 adrenergic agonist.

Indications. shock with sepsis, decreased SVR, elevated CO, hypotension.

Dose. 1-20 mcg/min.

Standard conc. 4 mg/250 cc; 15 cc/hr = 4 mcg/min.

Adverse effects. Ischemic necrosis and sloughing of superficial tissues will result if extravasation occurs, hypertension, arrhythmias, myocardial ischemia, increased uterine contractility, constricted microcirculation.

Octreotide (Sandostatin)

Actions. Somatostatin analogue that suppresses release of serotonin, gastrin, vasoactive intestinal peptide, insulin, glucagon and secretin.

Indications. Relief of flushing, bronchospasm, hypotension from carcinoid

tumor.
Dose. 50 mcg IV/SQ prn.
Adverse effects. May cause nausea, decreased gastrointestinal tract motility, transient hyperglycemia.

Ondansetron (Zofran)
Actions. Serotonin receptor selective antiemetic.
Indications. Prevention of postoperative nausea and/or vomiting.
Adult dose. 4 mg undiluted IV in not less than 30 seconds.
Pediatric dose. 0.05-0.075 mg/kg IV in not less than 30 seconds.
Adverse effects. Headache, dizziness, musculoskeletal pain, drowsiness, sedation, shivers, reversible transaminase elevation.

Oxytocin (Pitocin)
Actions. Reduced postpartum blood loss by contraction of uterine smooth muscle. Renal, coronary, and cerebral vasodilation.
Indications. Postpartum hemorrhage, uterine atony, augmentation of labor.
Dose. Uterine atony: 10-40 units in 1000 cc crystalloid; labor induction: 0.0005 -0.002 units/min.
Adverse effects. May cause uterine tetany and rupture, fetal distress. IV bolus can cause hypotension, tachycardia, dysrhythmia.

Phenylephrine (Neo-Synephrine)
Actions. Alpha adrenergic agonist (direct).
Indications. Hypotension.
Dose. 50-200 mcg bolus or 20-100 mcg/min continuous infusion.
Standard conc. For bolus 50 mcg/cc; for infusion 40-100 mcg/cc.
Adverse effects. Hypertension, reflex bradycardia.

Physostigmine (Antilirium)
Actions. Inhibition of cholinesterase, central and peripheral cholinergic effects.
Indications. Postoperative delirium, tricyclic antidepressant overdose, reversal of CNS effects of anticholinergic drugs.
Dose. 0.5-2.0 mg IV q15 minutes.
Adverse effects. May cause bradycardia, tremor, convulsions, hallucinations, psychiatric or CNS depression, mild ganglionic blockade, cholinergic crisis.

Procainamide (Pronestyl)
Actions. Antiarrhythmic effect.
Indications. Atrial and ventricular arrhythmias.
Load. Continuous infusion of 20-30 mg/min until (1) arrhythmia suppressed; (2) hypotension ensues; (3) the QRS complex widened by 50%; or (4) a total of 1 gm or 17 mg/kg has been given.
Maintenance. 1-4 mg/min.
Standard concentration. 2 gm/500 cc D_5W: 30 cc/hr = 2 mg/min.
Therapeutic level. 4-10 mcg/mL.
Adverse effects. Hypotension, heart block, myocardial depression, ventricular dysrhythmias, lupus, fever, agranulocytosis, GI irritation.

Propofol
Action. Increases activity of inhibitory GABA synapses.
Indications. IV induction agent for general anesthesia.
Induction. 1.5-2.5 mg/kg; reduce w/age >50.
Maintenance. 0.1-0.2 mg/kg/min or 6-12 mg/kg/hr combined with nitrous oxide and opiate.
Sedation. 25-150 mcg/kg/min.
Adverse effects. May cause pain during administration. Pain is reduced by prior administration of opioids or lidocaine.

Promethazine (Phenergan)
Actions. Antagonist of H1, D2, and muscarinic receptors. Antiemetic and sedative.
Indications. Allergies, anaphylaxis, nausea and vomiting, sedation.
Dose. 12.5-50 mg IV q4-6 hr prn.
Adverse effects. May cause mild hypotension or mild anticholinergic effects. Crosses placenta. May interfere with blood grouping. Intraarterial injection can cause gangrene.

Prostaglandin E1 (Alprostadil)
Actions. Vascular smooth muscle and uterine smooth muscle relaxation.
Indications. Pulmonary vasodilator, maintenance of patent ductus arteriosus.
Standard concentration. 500 mcg (1 vial) in 99 cc D_5W (5 mcg/cc).
Dose. Start at 0.05 mcg/kg/min (0.01 cc/kg/min); may increase to as high as 0.5 mcg/kg/min.
Adverse effects. Hypotension, apnea, flushing, bradycardia.
Misc. Rapidly metabolized.

Protamine sulfate
Actions. Antagonist of heparin's anticoagulant effect.
Indications. Reversal of the effects of heparin.
Dose. 1-3 mg per 100 units heparin, maximum 50 mg over 10 minutes, given slowly. 1.3 mg/kg of protamine for each 100 units of heparin present as calculated from the ACT.
Adverse effects. Hypotension (rapid injection secondary to histamine release), pulmonary hypertension and allergic reactions (seen in patients receiving protamine containing insulin preparations and in some patients allergic to fish).

Ritodrine (Yutopar)
Actions. Beta-2 selective adrenergic agonist that decreases uterine contractility.
Indications. Tocolysis (inhibition of preterm labor)
Dose. IV infusion 0.1-0.35 mg/min.
Adverse effects. Dose related increases in maternal and fetal heart rate and blood pressure due to beta-1 stimulation. May cause pulmonary edema, insulin resistance, potentiation of dysrhythmias and hypotension by magnesium. Contraindicated in eclampsia, pulmonary hypertension, and hyperthyroidism.

Pharmacology

Terbutaline (Brethine)
Actions. Beta-1 selective adrenergic agonist.
Indications. Bronchospasm and tocolysis.
Dose. Bronchospasm (adult): 0.25 mg SQ; repeat in 15 min prn; (pediatric): 3.5-5.0 mcg/kg SQ. Tocolysis: 10 mcg/kg IV infusion up to 80 mcg/min
Adverse effects. May cause dysrhythmias, pulmonary edema, hypertension, hypokalemia, or CNS excitement.

Vasopressin (Pitressin)
Actions. Synthetic analogue of arginine vasopressin; antidiuretic. Produces contraction of the smooth muscle.
Indications. Diabetes insipidus, GI bleeding.
Standard conc. 200 units vasopressin in 250 cc D_5W or NS (0.8 units/mL)
Dose. GI hemorrhage: infusion of 0.2-0.9 units/min
Adverse effects. Cardiotoxicity (myocardial ischemia, bradycardia), abdominal cramps, nausea, diarrhea, bowel infarction, water intoxication.
Misc. Usually combined with nitroglycerin infusion to reverse cardiotoxic effects while reducing the increase in portal venous resistance.

Verapamil (Calan)
Actions. Blockade of calcium channels in heart. Prolongation of PR interval with negative inotropy and chronotropy. Systemic and coronary vasodilation.
Indications. Supraventricular tachycardia, atrial fibrillation or flutter, Wolff-Parkinson-White syndrome.
Dose (adult). 2.5 -10 mg (75-150 mcg/kg) IV over 2 minutes. If no response in 30 minutes, repeat 10 mg.
Dose (pediatric). 0.1-0.3 mg/kg IV, repeat once if no response in 30 minutes.
Adverse effects. May cause severe bradycardia, AV block, excessive hypotension, congestive heart failure. May increase ventricular response to atrial fibrillation or flutter in patients with accessory tracts.

Drip Rates
cc/hr = (mcg/kg/min x 60 x wt(kg))/mcg/cc
mcg/kg/min = [(cc/hr) x (mcg/cc)]/60 x wt(kg)

Commonly Used Antibiotics		
Drug	Adult IV Dose	Dose Interval
Ampicillin	1 gm	q4-8 hrs
Cefazolin	0.5-1.0 gm	q4-8 hrs
Cefotetan	1-2 gm	q12 hrs
Clindamycin	600 mg	q6-8 hrs
Erythromycin	0.5-1.0 gm	q6 hrs
Gentamicin	60-120 mg	q8-12 hr (over 20 min)

70 Pharmacology

Drug	Adult IV Dose	Dose Interval
Metronidazole	500 mg	q6 hrs (over 15 min)
Tobramycin	60-120 mg	q8 hrs
Vancomycin	0.5-1.0 gm	q6-8 hrs (over 30+ min)

Parenteral Treatment of Acute Hypertension

Agent	Dosage Range	Onset	Duration
Nitroprusside	0.5-10 mcg/kg/min	30-60 sec	1-5 min
Nitroglycerin	5-100 mcg/min	1 min	3-5 min
Esmolol	0.5 mg/kg over 1 min 50-300 mcg/kg/min	1 min	12-20 min
Labetalol	5-20 mg	1-2 min	4-8 hr
Trimethaphan	3-4 mg/min	1-3 min	10-30 min
Phentolamine	2.5-5 mg	1-10 min	20-40 min
Hydralazine	5-20 mg	5-20 min	4-8 hr
Methyldopa	250-1000 mg	2-3 hr	6-12 hr

Pharmacology of Antihypertensive Parenteral Agents

Drug	Site of Vasodilation	Advantages	Side Effects/Problems
Nitroprusside	Direct dilator (balanced)	Immediate action Easy to titrate No CNS effects	Hypotension Reflex tachycardia Cyanide toxicity Methemoglobin
Nitroglycerin	Direct dilator (venous > arterial)	Coronary dilator	Headache Absorbed into IV tubing ETOH vehicle
Hydralazine	Direct dilator arterial >> venous	No CNS effects	Reflex tach, Lupus, Local thrombophlebitis
Trimethaphan	Ganglionic blocker	Aortic aneurysm Subarachnoid bleed	Anticholinergic effects Decreased cardiac output
Phentolamine	Alpha blocker direct vasodilator	Pheochromocytoma MAO crisis	Reflex tachycardia Tachyphylaxis

Drug	Site of Vasodilation	Advantages	Side Effects/Problems
Labetalol	Alpha and beta blockers	No overshoot hypotension Maintained CO, HR	Exacerbation of CHF, asthma, AV block, bronchospasm

Cardiovascular Physiology

Cardiopulmonary/Hemodynamic Parameters

Parameter	Formula	Normal Range
RA, CVP		2-10 mmHg
LA or LVEDP		4-12
RV		15-30/0-5 mmHg
PAS/ PAD		15-30/8-15 mmHg
MPAP	PAD + (PAS-PAD/3) or [(PAD)2 + PAS]/3	10-18 mmHg
PCWP		5-16 mmHg
MAP	DBP + (SBP-DBP/3) or [(DBP)2 + SBP]/3	75-110 mmHg
SVR	(MAP-CVP x 79.9)/CO	770-1500 dynes/sec/cm5
PVR	(MPAP-PCWP x 79.9)/CO	20-120 dynes/sec/cm5
CaO_2	(Hgbx1.34)SaO_2+(PaO_2x 0.0031)	16-22 mL O_2/dL blood
CvO_2	(Hgbx1.34)SvO_2+(PaO_2x 0.0031)	12-77 mL O_2/dL blood
$C(a-v)O_2$	(Hb x 1.34)(SaO_2 - SvO_2)	3.5-5.5 mL O_2/dL blood
SV	CO x 1000/HR	60-100 mL
CO	SV x HR=VO_2/C(a-v)O_2x10	3-9 liters/min
CI	CO/body surface area	2.1-4.9 L/min/m2
DO_2	CaO_2 x CO x 10	700-1400 mL/min
PAO_2	FIO_2 x (PB-PH_2O)-($PaCO_2$/0.8)	
A-a gradient	[(713)FIO_2-$PaCO_2$ (1.25)]-PaO_2	2-22 mmHg (RA)
Qs/Qt	(CcO_2-CaO_2)/(CcO_2-CvO_2)	0.05 or less
Creatinine Clearance	(Urine Cr/Serum Cr) x 70	Male=125; Female=105
Fractional Excretion of Sodium	(Ur Na/Plasma Na)/(Ur Cr/Pl Cr) x 100	pre-renal <1; ATN>1
PaO_2	102-(age/3)	

Cardiovascular Physiology

Parameter	Formula	Normal Range
Coronary Perfusion Pressure (CPP)	Art Diastolic BP - LVEDP	
SvO_2	$SaO_2 - VO_2/(CO \times Hb)(13.4)$	68-77%
VO_2	$Hb \times 1.34 \times CO \times 10 \times (SaO_2 - SvO_2)$	
Fick equation (VO_2)	$CO \times C(a-v)O_2$	225-275 mL/min
Body Mass Index (BMI)	$wt\,(kg)/ht\,(m)^2$	Obese >28 Morbidly obese >35
V_D/V_T	$(PaCO_2 - P_ECO_2)/PaCO_2$	Normal: 33%.

Cardiovascular Agents: Systemic Effects

Drug	CO	PCWP	SVR	MAP	HR	CVP	PVR
Norepinephrine	I	I	I	I	NC	I	I
Phenylephrine	D	I	I	I	D	I	I
Epinephrine	I	I	I	I	I	I	I
Dobutamine	II	D	D	I	I	D	D
Dopamine <6 mcg/kg/min	I	I	I	I	I	I	NC
Dopamine >6 mcg/kg/min	I	II	II	II	I	II	I
Digoxin	I	NC	NC	NC	D	NC	NC
Isoproterenol	II	D	D	D	II	D	D
Amrinone	I	D	D	NC	I	D	D
Nitroglycerin 20-40 mcg/min	NC	D	NC	NC	NC	D	NC
Nitroglycerin 50-250 mcg/min	I	D	D	D	I	D	D
Nitroprusside	I	D	D	D	I	D	D

Key: I=Increased; II=Large Increase; D=Decreased; NC=No Change

74 Cardiovascular Physiology

Adrenergic Agonists: System Effects

Drug	HR	MAP	CO	PVR	Broncho-dilation	Renal BF
Phenylephrine	-	+++	-	+++	0	---
Methyldopa	-	--	-	--	0	+
Epinephrine	++	+	++	-/+	++	--
Ephedrine	++	++	++	+	++	--
Norepinephrine	-	+++	-/+	+++	0	---
Dopamine	+/++	+	+++	+	0	+++
Isoproterenol	+++	-	+++	--	+++	-/+
Dobutamine	+	+	+++	-	0	+

Key: O = No effect; + = Minimal effect; ++ = Moderate effect; +++ = Marked effect. HR = heart rate; MAP = mean arterial pressure; CO = cardiac output; PVR = pulmonary vascular resistance; BF = blood flow.

Electrocardiograms

Interpretation format	Normal intervals (each small block=0.04 sec)		
1. Rate	P-R: 0.12-0.20 msec	Q-T (msec)	HR (bpm)
2. Rhythm	QRS: 0.06-0.10 msec	0.33-0.43	60
3. Intervals		0.31-0.41	70
4. Axis		0.29-0.38	80
5. Hypertrophy		0.28-0.36	90
6. Infarction/ischemia		0.27-0.35	100
7. Ectopy			

Cardiovascular Physiology

Electrolyte Abnormalities On EKG	
Hyperkalemia	Tall peaked T waves QRS widening ST elevation Loss of P waves
Hypokalemia	Small T wave/U wave QRS widening ST depression
Hypercalcemia	Shortening of QTc
Hypocalcemia	Prolongation of QTc

Localization of myocardial infarction

Location of MI	Q wave or ST change	Reciprocal ST depress
Anterior	V2-V4 (also poor R wave	II, III, AVF
	progression V1-V6)	
Antero-Septal	V1-V3	
Antero-Lateral	I, aVL, V4-V6	
Lateral	I, AVL, V5-V6	V1, V3
Inferior	II, III, AVF	I, AVL
Posterior	Tall R/T waves V1-V3	V1-V3
Subendocardial	ST depression in ant leads or inferior leads	

(Q wave >0.04 sec and >25% the height of the R wave)

LVH criteria
RV5 or RV6 >26 mm
SV1 or SV2 + RV5
  or RV6 >35 mm
R I +S III >25 mm
RaVL >13 mm
RaVF >20 mm

RVH criteria
R>S in V1 or V3
qR in V1 or V3
RAD
Wide QRS

Atrial hypertrophy
RAH: diphasic P with tall
  initial component
LAH: diphasic P with
  persistent S in V4-V6
  wide terminal component

Bundle branch block (QRS >0.12 sec)

Left BBB
Absence of septal Q waves in
  V4-V6, I, AVL
RR' or M pattern of QRS in
  I, aVL, V4-V6
2° ST, T wave change I, aVL, V4-V6

Right BBB
RR' or M pattern of QRS
  in V1-V3
Deep/round S waves in I, aVL,
  V4-V6
2° ST, T wave change in V1-V3

Atrioventricular Heart Blocks

I. First degree heart block: PR interval >0.20 sec.
II. Second degree heart block
   A. Mobitz Type I (Wenckebach): PR interval increases until QRS dropped, delta wave.

B. Mobitz Type II (infra His) PR interval constant until QRS dropped.

III. Third degree heart block: No AV conduction (P has no relation to QRS).

Electrocardiogram Changes

I. Prolonged QT Interval: hypocalcemia, hypokalemia, hypomagnesemia, acute MI, acute myocarditis, procainamide, quinidine, tricyclics.
II. Shortened QT Interval: hypercalcemia, digitalis.
III. LAD: LVH, left ant hemiblock, inferior wall MI.
IV. RAD: RVH, left post hemiblock, dextrocardia, pulmonary infarct, RBBB, lateral MI.
V. Pericarditis: diffuse ST elevation concave upward and/or diffuse PR depression and/or diffuse T wave inversion.
VI. Digitalis toxicity: ventricular arrhythmias, conduction abnormalities.
VII. Quinidine/procainamide: prolonged QT, flattened T wave, QRS widening.
VIII. Hypothermia: bradycardia, AV junctional, elevated J point, prolong QT.
IX. Orthotopic heart transplantation: the patient's original SA node often remains with the original atria, therefore, two P waves can be seen.
X. Head injuries: dysrhythmias and electrocardiographic abnormalities in the T wave, U wave, ST segment, and QT interval are common following head injuries but are not necessarily associated with cardiac injury; they likely represent altered autonomic function.

Electrocardiographic Detection of Perioperative Myocardial Ischemia

I. Single lead EKG sensitivity: V5 (75%), V4 (61%), V6 (37%), V3 (33%), II (24%), and all others <14%.
II. Combination leads: leads II and V5 increase sensitivity to 85%, leads V4 and V5 increase sensitivity to 90%, increasing to 96% by combining II, V4, and V5, and to 100% when five leads were used (V2-V5 and II).

Pacemakers

Pacemakers: Nomenclature For Description Of Pacemaker Function				
First letter: chamber paced	**Second letter: chamber sensed**	**Third letter: generator response**	**Fourth letter: program functions**	**Fifth letter: antitachycardia functions**
V-Ventricle	V-Ventricle	T-Triggered	P-Program[2]	B-Bursts
A-Atrium	A-Atrium	I-Inhibited	M-Multi-program	N-Normal rate competition[4]
D-Dual chamber	D-Dual chamber	D-Dual chamber	C-Communicating	S-Scanning[5]

Cardiovascular Physiology 77

First letter: chamber paced	Second letter: chamber sensed	Third letter: generator response	Fourth letter: program functions	Fifth letter: antitachy-cardia functions
	O-None (Asynchronous)	O-None (Asynchronous)	O-None (fixed function)	E-External[6]
		R-Reverse Functions[1]		

1. Pacemaker activated at fast rates only (ie, upon sensing a tachyarrhythmia as opposed to bradyarrhythmia).
2. Rate and/or output only.
3. Telemetry, interrogation (P or M implicit).
4. Paces at normal rate upon sensing tachyarrhythmia (underdrive pacing).
5. Scanning response (such as time extrasystoles).
6. External control (activated by a magnet, radiofrequency, or other means).

I. Preoperative pacemaker evaluation
   A. Determine the indications for the pacemaker.
   B. Determine type of generator, date placed, and the preset rate.
   C. Define pacemaker function.
   D. The patient should be questioned for history of vertigo, syncope, light headedness, or return of any pre-pacemaker symptoms which may reflect dysfunction of the pacemaker.
   E. Laboratory: Serum electrolytes (hypokalemia can increase the negative cell membrane potential increasing threshold for pacemaker to capture).
   F. Chest x-ray: Looking for a dislodged electrode or fracture, and the make and model, if available.

II. Intraoperative management
   A. The grounding pad for the electrocautery should be placed as far away from pulse generator as possible.
   B. Monitor heart rate during electrocautery with a stethoscope, pulse oximetry, or arterial line.
   C. A magnet placed over the pulse generator will convert a demand (VVI) pacemaker into an asynchronous (VOO) pacemaker.

III. Indications for temporary pacemaker
   A. Symptomatic sick sinus syndrome.
   B. Symptomatic hypertensive carotid sinus syndrome with cardio-inhibitory (not just vasodepressor) response.
   C. Mobitz type 2 block.
   D. Acute MI with RBBB or LBBB.
   E. Comatose trauma patient with bifascicular block.
   F. Trifascicular block.
   G. Symptomatic beta blocker overdose.

Central Venous Pressure Monitoring

I. Indications for central venous pressure monitoring
   A. Major thoracic procedures involving large fluid shifts or blood losses in patients with good heart function.

78 Cardiovascular Physiology

- **B.** Intravascular volume assessment when urine output is unreliable or unavailable (eg, renal failure).
- **C.** Major trauma.
- **D.** Frequent blood sampling in patients not requiring an arterial line.
- **E.** Venous access for vasoactive or caustic drugs.
- **F.** Chronic drug administration
- **G.** Inadequate peripheral intravenous access.
- **H.** Rapid infusion of intravenous fluids using large cannulae.

Central Pressure Monitoring: Central Venous Pressure Waves

Component	EKG	Cardiac Cycle	Mechanical Event
a Wave	Follows P wave	End diastole	Atrial Contraction
c Wave	Follows the onset of the QRS	Early systole	Isovolumic ventricular contraction, tricuspid motion toward atrium
v Wave	Follows T wave	Late systole	Systolic filling of atrium
h Wave		Mid diastole	Mid-diastolic pressure plateau (occurs with slow heart rates and prolonged diastole)
x Descent		Midsystole	Atrial relaxation, descent of the base, systolic collapse
y Descent		Early diastole	Early ventricular filling, diastolic collapse

II. Respiratory influences
- **A. End expiration.** CVP measurements should be made at end expiration because pleural and pericardial pressures approach atmospheric pressure under these conditions.
- **B. Spontaneous ventilation.** During spontaneous breathing, inspiration causes a decrease in intrapleural pressure and juxtacardiac pressure, which is transmitted in part to the right atrium and produces a decrease in CVP.
- **C. Mechanical ventilation.** Positive-pressure ventilation causes intrathoracic and juxtacardiac pressure to increase during inspiration, producing a increase in CVP.
- **D. PEEP.** As intrathoracic pressure increases from added PEEP, CVP measurements increases. This may be associated with a reduction in transmural filling pressure, preload, and venous return.

III. CVP Abnormalities
- **A. Atrial fibrillation.** The a wave disappears, and the c wave becomes more prominent since atrial volume is greater at end-diastole. Fibrillation waves may be noticed in the CVP tracing.
- **B. Isorhythmic A-V dissociation or junctional rhythm.** Atrial contraction may occur against a closed tricuspid valve, resulting in a "cannon a wave."
- **C. Tricuspid regurgitation.** Causes "ventricularization" of the CVP trace, with a broad, tall systolic c-v wave that begins early in systole and

obliterates the x descent. Unlike a normal v wave, the c-v wave begins immediately after the QRS, leaving only a y descent.
- **D. Tricuspid stenosis.** Prominent a wave as the atrium contracts against a stenotic valve; the y descent following the v wave is obstructed.
- **E. Right ventricular ischemia and infarction**
  1. Diagnosis is suggested by arterial hypotension in combination with disproportionate elevation of the CVP as compared to the PCWP. Mean CVP may approach or exceed the mean PCWP.
  2. Elevated right ventricular filling pressure produces prominent a and v waves and steep x and y descents, giving the waveform an M or W configuration.
- **F. Pericardial constriction.** Central venous pressure is usually markedly elevated, and the trace resembles that seen with right ventricular infarction. prominent a and v waves and steep x and y descents, creating an M pattern. Often the steep y descent in early diastole is short lived, and the CVP in mid-diastole rises to a plateau until the a wave is inscribed at end-diastole (similar to the h wave).
- **G. Cardiac tamponade.** Venous pressure waveform becomes monophasic with a characteristic obliteration of the diastolic y descent. The y descent is obliterated because early diastolic runoff from atrium to ventricle is impaired by the compressive pericardial fluid collection.

Pulmonary Artery Catheterization

I. Common indications for pulmonary artery catheterization
A. Cardiac disease
1. Cardiac disease with left ventricular dysfunction or recent MI.
2. Valvular heart disease.
3. Heart failure.
B. Pulmonary disease
1. Acute respiratory failure.
2. Severe chronic obstructive pulmonary disease.
C. Fluid Management

Pulmonary Artery Catheter Distances (cm)			
Vein	Right Atrium	Right Ventricle	Pulmonary Artery
Internal Jugular Right Left	20 25	30 35	40 50
Subclavian	15	25	40
Antecubital Right Left	40 45	50 55	65 70

80 Cardiovascular Physiology

Vein	Right Atrium	Right Ventricle	Pulmonary Artery
Femoral	30	40	55

II. Contraindications
A. Absolute contraindications
1. Tricuspid or pulmonic valvular stenosis.
2. Right atrial or right ventricular masses (eg, tumor, clot).
3. Tetralogy or Fallot.

B. Relative contraindications
1. Severe dysrhythmias. Complete left bundle branch block (because of the risk of complete heart block), Wolff-Parkinson-White syndrome, and Ebstein's malformation (because of possible tachyarrhythmias).
2. Coagulopathy.
3. Newly inserted pacemaker wires.

III. Correct position
can be confirmed by a chest radiograph. Although most catheters migrate caudally and to the right side, occasionally a catheter will wedge anterior to the vena cava. In this position, true pulmonary capillary pressures may be less than alveolar pressures, resulting in spuriously elevated measurements during positive pressure ventilation.

IV. Indicators of proper tip placement include
A. A decline in pressure as the catheter moves from the pulmonary artery into the "wedged" position.
B. Ability to aspirate blood from the distal port (eliminating the possibility of overwedging).
C. A decline in end-tidal CO_2 concentration with inflation of the balloon (produced by a rise in alveolar dead space).

V. Complications
A. Endobronchial hemorrhage.
The incidence of pulmonary artery catheter-induced endobronchial hemorrhage is 0.06%-0.20%. Risk factors include advanced age, female sex, pulmonary hypertension, mitral stenosis, coagulopathy, distal placement of the catheter, and balloon hyperinflation.

B. Pulmonary infarction

VI. Conditions resulting in discrepancy between PCWP and LVEDP
A. Overestimating (PCWP > LVEDP)
1. Positive pressure ventilation
2. PEEP
3. Increased intrathoracic pressure
4. Non-zone III PAC placement
5. COPD
6. Tachycardia
7. Increased pulmonary vascular resistance
8. Mitral valve obstruction (stenosis, myxoma, clot)
9. Pulmonary venous compression (tumor, fibrosis)
10. Mitral regurgitation
11. Left-to-right intracardiac shunt

B. Conditions Causing Underestimating (PCWP < LVEDP)
1. Noncompliant left ventricle
2. Aortic regurgitation

Cardiovascular Physiology 81

3. Reduced pulmonary arterial tree (pneumonectomy, PE)

Chest Radiography

I. **Endotracheal tube position**. When the head is in the neutral position, the tip of the ET tube should rest at the mid-trachea level, 5 cm above the carina. In adult patients the T5-T7 vertebral level is a good estimate of carinal position if it cannot be directly visualized.

II. **Central venous catheters**
 A. The desirable location is in the mid-superior vena cava, with the tip directed inferiorly.
 B. The catheter's tip should not be allowed to migrate into the heart.

III. **Pulmonary artery catheters**
 A. The tip of the pulmonary artery catheter should rest below the level of the left atrium (zone 3) to reduce or eliminate transmission of alveolar pressure to the capillaries.
 B. With an uninflated balloon, the tip of the pulmonary artery catheter should overlie the middle third of the well-centered AP chest x-ray (within 5 cm of the midline). Distal migration is common in the first hours after insertion as the catheter softens and loses slack.

IV. **Intraaortic balloon pump (IABP).** Diastolic inflation of the balloon produces a distinct, rounded lucence within the aortic shadow, but in systole the deflated balloon is not visible. Ideal positioning places the catheter tip just distal to the left subclavian artery.

Mixed Venous Oxygen Saturation (SvO_2)

I. **Physiology.** SvO_2 is approximately equal to $SaO_2 - (VO_2/CO \times Hb)$. Normal range: 68-77%.

II. **Main factors** affecting SvO_2 are cardiac output, hemoglobin level, oxygen consumption (VO_2), and SaO_2.

III. **Causes of increased SvO_2**
 A. The most common cause is a permanently wedged catheter.
 B. Low VO_2 as seen with cyanide toxicity, carbon monoxide poisoning, increases in methemoglobin, sepsis, and hypothermia.
 C. High cardiac output, as seen with sepsis, burns, left to right shunts, atrioventricular fistulas, inotropic excess, hepatitis, and pancreatitis.
 D. High SaO_2 and high hemoglobin are not common causes.

IV. **Causes of decreased SvO_2**
 A. Decreased Hb.
 B. Increased VO_2 with fever, exercise, agitation, shivering or thyrotoxicosis.
 C. Low SaO_2 with hypoxia, respiratory distress syndrome, or inappropriate ventilatory changes.
 D. Low cardiac output as seen in myocardial infarction, CHF, or hypovolemia.

V. **Pitfalls in continuous venous oximetry**
 A. The most common errors in the continuous measurement of SvO_2 are calibration and catheter malposition. Distal migration of the PA catheter can cause an artifactually high oxygen saturation owing to highly

saturated pulmonary capillary blood being analyzed.
- **B.** The light intensity signal may decrease if there is fibrin or deposition over the fiberoptic bundles, or if the catheter tip is lodged against a vessel wall or bifurcation.
- **C.** Large fluctuations in the light intensity may indicate an intravascular volume deficit which allows compression or collapse of the pulmonary vasculature (especially during positive pressure ventilation).
- **D.** Causes of pulse oximetry artifact include (1) excessive ambient light; (2) motion; (3) methylene blue dye; (4) venous pulsations in a dependent limb; (5) low perfusion; and (6) optical shunting.

Respiratory Physiology

Pulmonary Function Tests

I. **Predicted vital capacity**
   A. Women. (21.78 - [0.101 x age in years]) x height in cm.
   B. Men. (27.63 - [0.112 x age in years]) x height in cm.
II. **PFTs associated with increased pulmonary morbidity**
   A. FEV_1 < 2 liters.
   B. FEV_1/FVC < 0.5.
   C. Vital capacity < 15 mL/kg.
   D. Maximum breathing capacity < 50% of predicted.

Pulmonary Function Tests							
Condition	Vital Capacity*	FEV_1*	Max Vol Vent*	Residual Vol*	DLCO✝	PaO_2	$PaCO_2$
Normal	>80	>75	>80	80-120	25-30	80-100	38-42
Restrictive							
Mild	60-80	>75	>80	80-120	-	nl	nl
Moderate	50-60	>75	>80	70-80	--	-	-
Severe	35-50	>75	60-80	60-70	---	-	-
Very	<35	>75	<60	<60	---	--	+
Obstructive							
Mild	>80	60-75	65-80	120-150	nl	-	nl
Moderate	>80	40-60	45-65	150-175	nl	--	-
Severe	-	<40	30-45	>200	-	--	+
Very	-	<40	<30	>200	-	---	++

*Percent predicted; **Percent vital capacity; ✝ mL/min/mmHg; - = Decrease; + = Increase

Hemoglobin Dissociation Curve

I. **Factors shifting the curve to the right** (decreasing Hb affinity for oxygen).
   A. Increasing hydrogen ion concentration (decreased pH).
   B. Increased 2,3-DPG concentration.
   C. Increased body temperature.
II. P_{50} (oxygen tension at which hemoglobin is 50% saturated)
   A. Normal adult hemoglobin. 26 mmHg.
   B. Fetal hemoglobin. 19 mmHg.
   C. Parturient maternal hemoglobin. 30 mmHg.
   D. Sickle hemoglobin. 31 mmHg.
   E. Erythrocytes stored for 28 days at 1-6 °C. 17 mmHg.

84 Respiratory Physiology

Pediatric vs Adult Respiratory Physiology		
Respiratory Parameter	**Neonate**	**Adult**
Tidal volume (normal)	6 cc/kg	6 cc/kg
Tidal volume (ventilated)	8-15 cc/kg	8-15 cc/kg
Dead space	2 cc/kg	2 cc/kg
Functional residual capacity	28 cc/kg	30-35 cc/kg
Oxygen consumption	5-6 cc/kg/min	2-3 cc/kg/min
Alveolar ventilation	100-150 cc/kg	50-60 cc/kg
VA/FRC	4.5:1	1.5:1
Closing volume	Increased	

Normal Respiratory Parameters			
Parameter	**Normal Range**	**Parameter**	**Normal Range**
Tidal Volume (VT) (spontaneous ventilation)	6 cc/kg	FRC-adults FRC-peds	32 cc/kg 34 cc/kg
Tidal Volume (mechanical ventilation)	8-15 cc/kg	O_2 Consumption (VO_2)	3-4 cc/kg adults 6-8 cc/kg neo/infant
Vital Capacity (VC)	60-70 cc/kg	Dead Space (VD)	2 cc/kg
VD/VT	33%	FEV1/FVC	>75%
Minute ventilation	80 cc/kg		

Oxygenation and Ventilation

I. Major causes of hypoxemia
   A. Low inspired oxygen concentration (decreased FiO_2).
   B. Hypoventilation.
   C. Shunt (normal shunt about 2%). hypoxemia caused by shunt cannot be

overcome by increasing the inspired oxygen concentration.
   D. Ventilation perfusion (V/Q) mismatch. common causes of V/Q mismatch are atelectasis, patient positioning, bronchial intubation, one-lung ventilation, bronchospasm, pneumonia, mucus plugging, acute respiratory distress syndrome (ARDS) and airway obstruction.
   E. Diffusion abnormalities.
   F. Cardiac output - oxygen carrying capacity abnormalities (CO/O_2 capacity). as cardiac output or oxygen carrying capacity decrease, oxygen delivery will decrease resulting in hypoxemia.

II. Causes of hypercarbia
   A. Hypoventilation. Common causes include muscle paralysis, inadequate mechanical ventilation, inhalational anesthetics, and narcotics.
   B. Increased CO_2 production. Including malignant hyperthermia, fever, and thyrotoxicosis.
   C. Iatrogenic. Common examples include sodium bicarbonate administration and depletion of the CO_2 absorbent.

III. **Methods to improve oxygenation**
   A. Increased FiO2.
   B. Increase minute ventilation.
   C. Increase cardiac output (and increase oxygen delivery to tissues).
   D. Increase oxygen carrying capacity (hemoglobin).
   E. Optimize V/Q relationships.
   F. Cardiopulmonary bypass. Decrease oxygen consumption from pain, shivering, or fever.

Arterial Blood Gases

I. Golden rules of ABGs
   A. $PaCO_2$ change of 10 corresponds to a pH change of 0.08.
   B. $PaCO_2$ increases HCO_3 concentration. initially by 1; chronically by 3.
   C. $PaCO_2$ decreases HCO_3 concentration. initially by 2; chronically by 5.
   D. pH change of 0.15 corresponds to BE change of 10 mEq/l.

Arterial Blood Gases (Normal Values)						
	Newborn	1-24 months	7-19 yrs	Adult	Mixed Venous	Venous
pH	7.37	7.40	7.39	7.37-7.44	7.31-7.41	7.31- 7.41
PaO_2	15	90	96	80-100	35-40	30-50
$PaCO_2$	33	34	37	35-45	41-51	40-52
O_2 Sat (%)				>95	60-80	60-85
HCO_3	20	20	22	22-26	22-26	22-28

II. **Total body bicarbonate deficit** = base deficit (mEq/L) x patient wt (kg) x 0.4.
III. **Bicarbonate deficit** (HCO_3 deficit) = (total body water) x (24 - HCO_3).
IV. **Base excess (BE)** or deficit
   A. BE = HCO_3 + 10(pH - 7.40) - 24.
   B. Base excess or deficit is a calculated value that gives an estimation of "acid load."
   C. Negative values of base excess (ie, deficit) represent metabolic acidosis, and positive values indicated metabolic alkalosis.
V. **During apnea**, $PaCO_2$ increases 5-6 during the first minute and 3-4 for every minute thereafter.
VI. **Henderson-Hasselbach equation**
   A. pH = 6.1 + log[(HCO_3)/(0.03 x $PaCO_2$)]
   B. Modified equation. (H+) = [24 x pCO_2] / HCO_3
   C. pH = pk + log A-/HA
VII. **PaO_2 age adjustment**: PaO_2 = 102 - (age/3)

Saturation by PaO_2

100% = 90-100	90% = 60	75% = 40	60% = 30	30% = 20
95% = 70	80% = 50	70% = 35	50% = 27	

Anion Gap

Anion gap = Na - (Cl + HCO_3)   Normal anion gap = 8-16 mEq/l

Causes of Metabolic Acidosis

Increased anion gap (S.L.U.M.P.E.D.)
- **S**alicylates
- **L**actate
- **U**remic toxins
- **M**ethanol
- **P**araldehyde
- **E**thanol/ethylene glycol
- **D**iabetic ketoacidosis

Normal anion gap
- Renal causes
- Renal tubular acidosis
- Carbonic anhydrase inhibitors
- Lysine or arginine HCl
- GI bicarbonate loss
- Diarrhea
- Pancreatic fistula
- Ureterosigmoidostomy
- Addition of HCl
- Ammonium chloride

Airway Management

I. Airway innervation
A. Nasal mucosa. Sphenopalatine ganglion a branch of the middle division of cranial nerve V (trigeminal Nerve). The ganglion is located on the lateral wall posterior to the middle turbinate.
B. Uvula, tonsils, superior pharynx. Innervated by continued branches from the sphenopalatine ganglion.
C. Oral pharynx and supraglottic area. Innervated by branches of CN IX (glossopharyngeal nerve). These branches include lingual, pharyngeal, and tonsillar nerves.
D. Larynx. Sensory and motor is from the Vagus (CN X).
  1. **Sensory.** Above the vocal folds innervated by the internal branch of the superior laryngeal nerve; below the vocal folds innervated by the recurrent laryngeal nerve.
  2. **Motor.** All muscles are supplied by the recurrent laryngeal nerve except for the cricothyroid muscle which is supplied by the external branch of the superior laryngeal nerve.
E. Trachea. Innervated by the recurrent laryngeal nerve.

II. General preparation
A. Consider premedicating with either atropine or glycopyrrolate (to help decrease secretions) and/or sedation.
B. If considering a nasal intubation, give 4 drops of 0.25% Norsynephrine to each nare to help minimize bleeding. Other vasoconstrictors include oxymetazoline (Afrin) and cocaine.

Topical Nsal Agents For Nasal Intubation

Local Anesthetic	Concentration	Max Dose (mg/kg)
Cocaine	4-10%	3
Tetracaine	0.5-2%	1
Hexylcaine (Cyclaine)	5%	3
Lidocaine	2-4%	3
Dyclonine (Dyclone)	0.5%	4 (patients allergic to LA)

III. Nerve blocks
A. Nasotracheal nerve blocks
  1. **Sphenopalatine ganglion (nasal mucosa)**
     a. Cotton pledgets soaked with anesthetic solution (usually 20% benzocaine or 4% lidocaine) are placed in the nasal cavity at a 30 degree cephalad angulation to follow the middle turbinate back to the mucosa overlying the sphenoid bone.
     b. A second set of pledgets is introduced through the nares and passed along the turbinates to the posterior end of the nasal passage.

c. The pledgets should be left in place for at least 2-3 minutes to allow adequate diffusion of local anesthetic.
  2. **Lesser and pharyngeal palatine nerves**
     a. Landmarks. 1 cm medial to the third maxillary molar and 1 cm anterior to the junction of the hard and soft palates (usually 0.5 cm in diameter).
     b. Place a cotton pledget soaked with anesthetic solution on this site and wait 1 minute (provides topical anesthesia).
     c. Using a 25 g spinal needle create a 90 degree bend 3 cm from the tip. Probe the mucosa with the needle to find the a palatine foramen (usually up to 3), angulate the needle 15 degrees medially and advance 3 cm up the canal. After negative aspiration, inject 1-3 cc of 1-2% lidocaine with epinephrine.
 B. **Orotracheal nerve blocks**
  1. **Glossopharyngeal nerve.** Insert a 25 g spinal needle into the base of the posterior tonsillar pillar. After negative aspiration, inject 2-3 cc of 1-2% lidocaine with epinephrine. Repeat block on opposite side.
  2. **Superior laryngeal nerve**
     a. Place the patient supine with the neck extended.
     b. Find the thyrohyoid membrane (a soft depression between the hyoid and thyroid bones) and displace the hyoid bone laterally toward the side to be blocked.
     c. Insert a 25 g needle off the greater cornu of the hyoid bone, inferiorly, and advance 2-3 mm. As the needle passes through the thyrohyoid membrane, a slight loss of resistance is felt. Inject 2-3 cc of 1-2 % lidocaine with epinephrine. Repeat the block on opposite side.
  3. **Translaryngeal (transtracheal) nerve block**
     a. Landmarks. Cricothyroid membrane (located between the thyroid cartilage superiorly and the cricoid cartilage inferiorly).
     b. Insert a 20 g Angiocath, bevel up, at the upper edge of cricoid cartilage in the midline. Aspirate for air to confirm placement into the trachea. Remove the needle, leaving only the angio-catheter. Inject 3-5 cc of 2-4% lidocaine solution at end inspiration. This will usually result in a vigorous cough.

V. Common indications for tracheal intubation
 A. Provide patent airway.
 B. Protection from aspiration from gastric contents.
 C. Facilitate positive-pressure ventilation.
 D. Operative position other than supine.
 E. Operative site near or involving the upper airway.
 F. Airway maintenance by mask is difficult.
 G. Disease involving the upper airway.
 H. One-lung ventilation.
 I. Altered level of consciousness.
 J. Tracheobronchial toilet.
 K. Severe pulmonary or multisystem injury.

VI. Complications of endotracheal intubation
 A. **Complications occurring during intubation**
  1. Aspiration.
  2. Dental damage (chip tooth).
  3. Laceration of the lips or gums.

4. Laryngeal injury.
5. Esophageal intubation.
6. Endobronchial intubation.
7. Activation of the sympathetic nervous system (high blood pressure and tachycardia).
8. Bronchospasm.

B. **Complications occurring after extubation**
 1. Aspiration.
 2. Laryngospasm.
 3. Transient vocal cord incompetence.
 4. Glottic or subglottic edema.
 5. Pharyngitis or tracheitis.

Intubation Techniques

I. **Preparation for intubation**
  A. **Equipment.** Laryngoscope with working light, endotracheal tubes of appropriate sizes, malleable stylet, oxygen supply, suction with Yankauer tip, and functioning IV.
   1. **Laryngoscope blades**
      a. **Macintosh blade.** The Macintosh is a curved blade whose tip is inserted into the vallecula. Most adults require a Macintosh number 3 blade.
      b. **Miller blade.** The Miller is a straight blade that is passed so that the tip of the blade lies beneath the laryngeal surface of the epiglottis. The epiglottis is then lifted to expose the vocal cords. Most adults require a Miller number 3 blade.
  B. **Position** bed height to bring patient's head to a mid-abdominal height.
  C. **Head position.** Place the head in the "sniffing" position if there is no cervical spine injury. The sniffing position is characterized by flexion of the cervical spine and extension of the head at the atlantooccipital joint.

II. **Orotracheal intubation**
  A. Position the patient's head as noted above.
  B. Hold the laryngoscope in the palm of the left hand and introduce the blade into the right side of the patient's mouth. Advance the blade posteriorly and toward the midline, sweeping the tongue to the left. Check that the lower lip is not caught between the lower incisors and the laryngoscope blade.
  C. When the epiglottis is in view, advance the tip of the laryngoscope blade into the vallecula if using a Macintosh blade or under the epiglottis if using a Miller blade. Check that the upper lip is not caught between the upper incisors and the laryngoscope blade.
  D. Lift the laryngoscope upward and forward, in the direction of the long axis of the handle, to bring the larynx into view. Do not use the upper incisors as a fulcrum for leverage because this action may damage the upper incisors and may push the larynx out of sight.
  E. The vocal cords should be visualized prior to endotracheal placement. Posteriorly, the vocal cords terminate in the arytenoid cartilages. The tube should be seen to pass between the cords, anterior to the arytenoids. Pass the endotracheal tube into the pharynx with the right hand from the right side of the mouth; it should pass without resistance through the

90 Airway Management

vocal cords. The endotracheal tube cuff should lie in the upper trachea but beyond the larynx.

   F. Once the endotracheal tube is in place, inflate the cuff, confirm endotracheal intubation and secure the endotracheal tube. In order to minimize the pressure transmitted to the tracheal mucosa, the cuff should be inflated with the least amount of air necessary to create a seal during positive pressure ventilation. For patients intubated outside the operating room, obtain a portable chest x-ray following intubation to confirm tube placement and bilateral lung expansion.

III. Nasotracheal intubation

   A. Topical cocaine (or other anesthetic method) and phenylephrine should be applied to the nasal passages.

   B. Generously lubricate the nare and endotracheal tube. The endotracheal tube should be advanced through the nose directly backward toward the nasopharynx. A loss of resistance marks the entry into the oropharynx.

   C. The laryngoscope and Magill forceps can be used to guide the endotracheal tube into the trachea under direct vision. For awake spontaneously breathing patients, the blind technique can be used. While listening for breath sounds at the proximal end of the endotracheal tube, advance the tube during inspiration. A cough followed by a deep breath, condensation in the tube from exhaled moisture, and loss of voice suggest tracheal entry. A fiberoptic bronchoscope can be utilized to direct the tube into the trachea.

Rapid Sequence Induction/Intubation

I. Indications. Patients who are at risk for aspiration (eg, history of recent meal, gastroesophageal reflux, pregnancy, trauma).

II. Method

   A. Nonparticulate antacids, H_2-blockers and metoclopramide may be used preoperatively to decrease the acidity and volume of gastric secretions.

   B. Equipment is similar to that for any intubation but commonly includes several endotracheal tubes with stylet and cuff-inflation syringe in place, assortment of laryngoscope blades, functioning suction, and a patent IV.

   C. Preoxygenate before induction. Four maximal breaths of 100% oxygen over 30 seconds is as effective as breathing 100% oxygen spontaneously for 3-5 minutes.

   D. Induction is accomplished with any induction agent. Just before administration of the induction agent, cricoid pressure (Sellick's maneuver) should be applied.

   E. Muscle relaxant is usually given to help facilitate intubation. Succinylcholine (1-1.5 mg/kg) is the relaxant of choice and should be given immediately after the induction agent. Once the induction agent and muscle relaxant are given, there should be no attempt to ventilate the patient by mask.

   F. Intubation should be performed as soon as jaw relaxation has occured.. Cricoid pressure should be maintained until confirmation of tracheal placement of the endotracheal tube has ben confirmed. If the first attempt to intubate fails, cricoid pressure should be maintained continuously during all subsequent maneuvers, while mask ventilation with 100% oxygen is administered.

Confirmation of Tracheal Intubation

I. Direct visualization of the endotracheal tube passing though the vocal cords.
II. Carbon dioxide in exhaled gases (documentation of end-tidal CO_2 in at least three consecutive breaths).
III. Bilateral breath sounds.
IV. Absence of air movement during epigastric auscultation.
V. Condensation (fogging) of water vapor in the tube during exhalation.
VI. Refilling of reservoir bag during exhalation.
VII. Maintenance of arterial oxygenation.
VIII. Chest x-ray. The tip of endotracheal tube should be between the carina and thoracic inlet or approximately at the level of the aortic notch or at the level of T5.

Transtracheal Ventilation

1. Transtracheal ventilation can be used as a temporizing measure if mask ventilation and oxygenation become inadequate.
2. Technique. a catheter (12- or 14-gauge) is connected to a jet-type ventilator, which in turn is connected to an oxygen source capable of delivering gas at a pressure around 50 psi, and inserted into the trachea through the cricothyroid membrane. The gas is delivered intermittently by a hand-held actuator. The duration of ventilation is best assessed by watching the rise and fall of the chest: an inspiratory to expiratory ratio of 1:4 seconds is recommended.
3. Oxygenation usually improves rapidly, however, retention of carbon dioxide may limit the duration of the technique's usefulness.

Extubation Criteria

1. NIF > -20 cm H_2O
2. RR < 30/min
3. TV > 5 cc/kg
4. VC > 10 cc/kg
5. PaO_2 > 65-70 mm (FIO_2 < 40%)
6. $PaCO_2$ < 50 mm
7. Resting Min Vent < 10 l/min
8. LOC stable or improving
9. TV/RR > 10
10. Qs/Qt < 20%
11. Pmep > +40 cm H_2O
12. Vd/Vt < 0.6

Endotracheal Tube And Laryngoscope Blade Sizes		
Age	**Size**	**Type**
Premature	2.5	Miller 0: neonate/premature
Neonate	3.0 - 3.5	Miller 1: up to 6 - 8 months
6 - 12 months	3.5 - 4.0	Wis-Hipple 1.5: 9 months- 2 yrs
12 - 20 months	4.0	Miller 2: 2.5 - 5.0 years
Over 20 months	4.0 + Age (yrs.)/4	Macintosh 2: child over 5 yrs
Adults (>14 years)	Female 6.5-8.5	Macintosh 3-4: adults
	Male 7.0-10.0	Miller 3: adults

Mechanical Ventilation

I. **Types of mechanical ventilators**
   A. **Time cycled.** The tidal volume is delivered and inspiration ends after a preset time interval.
   B. **Volume cycled.** The tidal volume is delivered and inspiration ends after a preset time interval.
   C. **Pressure cycled.** The tidal volume is delivered and inspiration ends when a preset volume is delivered.
II. **Modes of mechanical ventilation**
   A. **Intermittent positive-pressure ventilatory modes (IPPV)**
   B. **Controlled mechanical ventilation (CMV).** Mechanical breaths are delivered at a preset rate and tidal volume regardless of the patient's effort.
   C. **Assist-control ventilation (AC).** A preset minute ventilation is delivered regardless of the patient's effort. The ventilator senses each patient-initiated spontaneous breath and delivers a preset tidal volume as well.
   D. **Intermittent mandatory ventilation (IMV).** The ventilator provides tidal volume breaths at a preset fixed rate. In between ventilator-delivered breaths, the patient is able to breathe spontaneously at any rate, tidal volume, or pattern.
   E. **Synchronized intermittent mandatory ventilation (SIMV).** Similar to IMV, with the ventilatory breaths timed to coincide with spontaneous effort.
   F. **Continuous positive airway pressure (CPAP).** A preset level of positive airway pressure is maintained throughout the respiratory cycle. The patient must be spontaneously breathing.
   G. **Inspiratory pressure support ventilation (IPS).** A preset pressure is obtained when the patient initiates an inspiratory effort.
   H. **Pressure-controlled ventilation**
      1. Maximum airway pressure is set on the ventilator, and tidal volume becomes the dependent variable.
      2. The duration of inspiration is determined by setting either the inspiratory time or the I:E ratio. Tidal volume is the product of inspiratory flow and inspiratory time.
      3. The primary advantage of pressure-controlled ventilation is reduction in peak airway pressure and potential improvement of gas exchange.
   I. **High frequency ventilation**
      1. **High frequency positive pressure ventilation (HFPPV).** Similar to conventional ventilation, however, tidal volumes are very small, and cycling frequencies are very fast (60-300).
      2. **High frequency jet ventilation (HFJV).** A small diameter injecting catheter positioned in the central airway pulses gas along the luminal axis under high pressure at a rapid cycling rate.
   J. **Pressure-controlled inverse ratio ventilation (PC-IRV).** Set by choosing a prolonged inspiratory time such that the time spend during inspiration exceeds expiratory time.
III. **Positive end-expiratory pressure (PEEP)**
   A. **Function of PEEP.** PEEP increases oxygenation by maximizing the ventilation-perfusion relationship in the lung. PEEP does this by maximizing the FRC (functional residual capacity), keeping lung volumes greater than closing capacity, therefore maintaining airways open and functional.

B. Adverse effects of PEEP
1. Decreased cardiac output.
2. Hypotension.
3. Worsening hypoxia.
4. Barotrauma (pneumothorax).
5. Increased intracranial pressure.
6. Decreased urine output.

IV. Ventilator Settings
- **A. FIO_2.** Normally start with 40% otherwise use 90-100% until first ABG available (1% decrease in FIO_2 = decrease PaO_2 by 7).
- **B. PEEP.** Initially none; start with 5 cm H_2O and increase in 3-5 cm H_2O increments if PaO_2 less than 60 mmHg with FIO_2 > 50%; over 10 cm H_2O normally requires pulmonary artery catheter.
- **C. Rate.** Start at 10-14 (for infants start at 25-30).
- **D. Tidal volume.** 10-15 ml/kg (infants 8-12 ml/kg).
- **E. Mode.** IMV, SIMV, CPAP, A/C, PSV.

Oxygen Therapy

I. Nasal cannulas.
FIO_2 increases by 3-4%/liter of O_2 given (up 40-50%).

II. Masks
- **A. Simple mask.** Simple mask may deliver oxygen flow rates from 6-15 liters per minute providing FIO_2 of 0.35-0.65.
- **B. Venturi mask** (air entrainment mask). Delivers up to 50% FIO_2.
- **C. Partial rebreathing mask.** Simple mask with a valveless reservoir bag and exhalation ports. Can deliver up to 80% FIO_2.
- **D. Nonrebreathing mask.** Simple mask with reservoir bag and unidirectional valve. Can deliver up to 95% FIO_2.
- **E. Aerosol face tent.** Delivers oxygen form variable oxygen nebulizer over mouth and nose.

Laryngeal Mask Airway

I. Indications for LMA
- **A.** In place of a face mask or endotracheal tube in a spontaneously breathing anesthetized patient.
- **B.** In place of an endotracheal tube, when breathing is being controlled, as long as the inflation pressure is not more than 20 cm H_2O.
- **C.** To aid in the management of the difficult airway (ie, the LMA can be used as a guide for fiberoptic intubation).

II. Contraindications for LMA
- **A.** The LMA does not provide an airtight seal of the airway and, thus, does not protect against gastric regurgitation and pulmonary aspiration.
- **B.** When controlled ventilation is likely to require a high-inflation pressure of more than 20 cm H_2O.

III. Insertion of the LMA
- **A.** Propofol (2.5-3.0 mg/kg) is the agent of choice for LMA insertion. Propofol relaxes the jaw and pharyngeal muscles better than thiopental.
- **B.** The leading edge of the deflated cuff should be wrinkle-free and facing

94 Airway Management

      away from the aperture. Lubricate only the back side of the cuff with a water soluble lubricant.
- C. The LMA is held like a pencil and is inserted via the mouth blindly in the midline with concavity forward while pressing on the anterior shaft with the tip of the index finger toward the hard palate and guiding it toward the pharynx.
- D. When the upper esophageal sphincter is reached, a characteristic resistance is felt. The cuff is then inflated with air (the cuff should be inflated without holding the tube to enable the expanding cuff to find its correct position in the pharynx).
- E. When correctly placed, the black vertical line on the posterior aspect of the tube should always face directly backward, toward the head of the patient.
- F. The LMA should be left in place until the patient can open his mouth on command. During emergence, the patient should not be stimulated (ie, suctioned), and the cuff should not be deflated until the patient can open his mouth on command.

IV. Complications
- A. Possibility of regurgitation and pulmonary aspiration.
- B. Oral and pharyngeal mucosa injury during insertion of the LMA.
- C. Laryngospasm and coughing (may occur if the LMA is inserted in a lightly anesthetized patient).
- D. Negative pressure pulmonary edema after improper placement in spontaneously breathing patient.

| LMA Sizes (ETT= endotracheal tube; * = cuffed tube) ||||
Size	Patient	Cuff Vol (mL)	Largest ETT
1	Infant up to 6.5 kg	4	3.5
2	Infants/Children up to 20 kg	10	4.5
2.5	Children between 20 - 30 kg	15	5.0
3	Children/small adults over 30 kg	20	6.0*
4	Average adults	30	6.0*
5	Large adults greater than 80 kg	30	7.0*

Esophageal Tracheal Combitube

- I. **Uses.** Emergency airway control in the difficult airway. Available only in one adult size (age >15 years and height >5 feet).
- II. **Insertion**
  - A. With the head in the neutral position, insert the ETC, with gentle pressure, up to the black marks (teeth should be between black marks).
  - B. Inflate the first pilot balloon (blue cuff) with 100 cc. As the cuff is inflated,

the combitube will pop out 1 cm.
   C. Inflate the second pilot balloon (white cuff) with 10-15 cc.
III. **Placement**
   A. Ventilate via longer (blue) lumen.
   B. If breath sounds are present, the ETC is in the esophagus; ventilate.
   C. If no breath sounds are heard, change ventilation to shorter lumen #2 (clear) and recheck for breath sounds. If breath sounds are present, the ETC is in the trachea; continue to ventilate.
   D. If no breath sounds or breath sounds faint, attempt to improve seal by adding up to 60 cc to balloon number 1.
   E. If unable to ventilate, deflate both cuffs, pull back 3 cm and reinflate cuffs. Ventilate via blue lumen and check for breath sounds. If still no breath sounds, deflate cuffs, remove ETC and start algorithm over.
IV. **Contraindications**
   A. Height less than 5 feet (only one size currently available).
   B. Intact gag reflex intact (will not tolerate cuff).
   C. Presence of esophageal disease (potential for bleeding or rupture).
   D. Ingestion of caustic substances (potential for rupture).
   E. Upper airway obstruction (foreign body, glottic edema, epiglottis).
V. **Concerns**
   A. Potential for nasopharyngeal, oropharyngeal or tracheal mucosal damage or edema (particularly if left in for greater than 2-8 hours).
   B. Inability to suction tracheal secretions when in esophageal position.
   C. Only one size available; single use makes it expensive.

Bullard Laryngoscope

I. **Clinical Uses**
   A. The Bullard laryngoscope, functioning as an indirect fiberoptic laryngoscope, provides direct visualization of the vocal cords. It is available in both adult and pediatric sizes.
   B. The advantage of this laryngoscope is that it can be introduced into the oropharynx with minimal mouth opening (oral opening of 0.64 cm required) and the patient can remain in anatomical position.
   C. Preloading the intubating stylet involves lubricating the stylet and positioning the endotracheal tube so that the distal end of the stylet projects through the Murphy's eye of the endotracheal tube.
   D. The blade is then inserted into the mouth, with the handle in the horizontal plane, and rotated into the vertical plane allowing it to slide around the midline of the tongue and into the posterior pharynx. Gentle traction is applied against the posterior surface of the tongue to obtain visualization of the glottic aperture.
   E. With the stylet pointed directly at the glottic opening, the endotracheal tube is advanced under direct vision into the trachea.

Laboratory Values

CSF
Glucose	40-70 mg/dL
Total Protein	20-45 mg/dL
CSF Pressure	50-180 mm H$_2$O
Leukocytes	Total<4 per mm3
Lymph	60-70%
Mono	30-50%
Neutro	1-3%

Renal
Cr Clearance	
Males	125 mL/min
Females	105 mL/min
Ur Creat	1.0-1.6 g/d
Ur Protein	<0.15 g/d
Ur K	25-100 meg/d
Ur Na	100-260 meg/d

Chemical

Acid Phosphatase	0-5.5 U/L	CPK	25-145 U/L
Albumin	3.5-5.5 g/dL	Creatinine	0.4-1.5 mg/dL
Alk Phosphatase	30-120 U/L	Ferritin	15-200 ng/mL
Aminotransferases		Glucose	70-140 mg/dL
AST (SGOT)	0-35 U/L	Iron	80-180 mcg/dL
ALT (SGPT)	0-35 U/L	Iron-Binding	250-450 mcg/dL
Ammonia	80-110 mcg/dL	Iron-Sat	20-45
Amylase	60-80 U/L	LDH	25-100 U/L
Bilirubin	Lipase	49-220 U/L	
Total	0.3-1.0 mg/dL	Magnesium	1.6-2.6 mg/dL
Direct	0.1-0.3 mg/dL	Osmolality	285-295
Indirect	0.2-0.7 mg/dL	Phosphorus	2.5-4.5 mg/dL
Calcium	8.6-10.5 mg/dL	Protein	5.5-8.0 mEq/L
CO$_2$	22-30 mEq/L	Sodium	136-145 mEq/L
Chloride	98-106 mEq/L	Triglycerides	<60 mg/dL
Cholesterol		Urea nitro	10-20 mg/dL
Total (years)		Uric Acid	
<29	<200 mg/dL	Males	2.5-8.0 mg/dL
30-39	<225 mg/dL	Females	1.5-6.0 mg/dL
40-49	<245 mg/dL		
>50	<265 mg/dL		
HDL	30-90 mg/dL		
LDL	50-190 mg/dL		

Complete Blood Count

Male
	1 month	6-12 years	Adult
WBC	5.0-19.5	5.0-13.5	4.5-11.0
RBC	3.0-5.4	4.0-5.2	4.6-6.2
Hb	14.0-18.0	11.5-15.5	14.0-18.0
Hct	31-55	35-45	42-52
RDW			11.5-14.5

Female
	1 month	6-12 years	Adult
WBC	5.0-19.5	5.0-13.5	4.5-11.0
RBC	3.0-5.4	4.0-5.2	4.2-5.4
Hb	14.0-18.0	11.5-15.5	12.0-16.0
Hct	31-55	35-45	37-47
RDW			11.5-14.5

Fluid and Electrolyte Management

I. **Functional fluid compartments**
   A. **Total body water (TBW).** 60% (adult males) or 50% (adult females) of ideal body weight (IBW).
   B. **Intracellular fluid (ICF).** Comprises approximately 35% of IBW or 60% of TBW. Principal potassium containing space.
   C. **Extracellular fluid (ECF).** Accounts for 25% of IBW or 40% of TBW and is subdivided into interstitial fluid (ISF) and blood volume (BV; about 8% of TBW). Principal sodium containing space.

II. **Guidelines for intraoperative crystalloid fluid replacement**
   A. Insensible losses. 2 mL/kg/hr
   B. Minor trauma/surgery. 3-4 mL/kg/hr
   C. Moderate trauma/surgery. 5-6 mL/kg/hr
   D. Major trauma/surgery. 7-8 mL/kg/hr

III. **Maintenance fluid requirements**
   A. First 10 kg. 4 mL/kg/hr
   B. Second 10 kg. 2 mL/kg/hr
   C. >20 kg. 1 mL/kg/hr

IV. **Daily electrolyte requirements**
   A. Na: 2-3 mEq/kg/24 hours
   B. K: 1-2 mEq/kg/24 hours
   C. Cl: 2-3 mEq/kg/24 hours

V. **Determinants of perioperative fluid requirements.** Basal requirements, preoperative deficits, third-space losses, transcellular fluid losses, effects of anesthetic agents and technique.

VI. **Calculated osmolality** = 2 Na + glucose/18 + BUN/2.8 + ethanol/4.6 + isopropanol/6 + methanol/3.2 + ethylene glycol/6.2 (norm 280-295).

VII. **Calcium disturbances**
   A. Normal plasma concentration is 8.5-10.5 mg/dL with 50% free ionized 40% protein bound.
   B. Normal free ionized concentration is 4.5-5 mg/dL.
   C. Corrected calcium = measured calcium / [0.6 + (total protein / 8.5)].
   D. For each 1 gm/dL change in albumin there is a corresponding 0.8 mg/dL change in total calcium (free ionized calcium is not affected).
   E. Ionized calcium increases 0.16 mg/dL for each decrease of 0.1 unit in plasma pH.

VIII. **Glucose.** For each 100 mg/dL glucose above normal there is a corresponding fall in sodium by 1.6 mEq/l.

Fluids							
Fluid	Glu gm/L	Na	Cl	K	Ca	HCO$_3$	Kcal/L
D$_5$W	50						170
NS		154	154				
D5 1/4NS	50	38	38				170
LR		130	110	4	3	27	<10

Blood Therapy Management

- **Blood loss management**
    - **A. Estimated blood volume (EBV)**
        1. 100-120 mL/kg for premature infant
        2. 90 mL/kg for full-term infant
        3. 80 mL/kg for infants 3 to 12 months
        4. 70 mL/kg thereafter
    - **B.** Replace every 1 mL blood loss with 3 mL crystalloid or 1 cc PRBC
    - **C. PRBC.** one unit PRC increases Hct about 3% and Hb about 1 g/dL
        1. 3 mL/kg PRC increases Hb about 1 g/dL
        2. 10 mL/kg PRBC increases Hct about 10%
    - **D. Max allowable blood loss**=[EBV x (Hct - target Hct)]/ Hct
    - **E. Fluid replacement equivalents**
        1. **Crystalloid.** 3 cc/1 cc estimated blood loss [EBL]
        2. **Colloid.** 1 cc/cc EBL
        3. **Whole blood.** 1 cc/cc EBL
        4. **Packed red blood cells.** ½ cc/cc EBL
- **I. Compatibility testing**
    - **A. Type specific.** ABO-Rh typing only; 99.80% compatible.
    - **B. Type and screen.** ABO-Rh and screen; 99.94% compatible.
    - **C. Type and crossmatch.** ABO-Rh, screen, and crossmatch; 99.95% compatible.
    - **D. Screening donor blood.** Hematocrit is determined, if normal, the blood is typed, screened for antibodies, and tested for hepatitis B, hepatitis C, syphilis, HIV-1, HIV-2, and human T-cell lymphotropic viurses I and II. ALT is also measured as a surrogate marker of nonspecific liver infection.
- **II. Blood component therapy**
    - **A. Whole blood.** 40% hematocrit; used primarily in hemorrhagic shock.
    - **B. Packed red blood cells (PRBC).** 70% hematocrit; each unit contains 250-300 mL volume and rises Hb approximately 1 g/dL.
    - **C. Platelets.** Single donor bag (10-25 mL/bag) or multiple donor bag (50-70 mL/bag); approximately 5.5×10^5 platelets per unit; each unit increases platelet count 5000-10000; platelets are the only blood product stored at room temperature.
    - **D. Fresh frozen plasma (FFP).** 250 cc/bag; contains 200 units of procoagulants and plasma proteins including factors V and VIII.
    - **E. Cryoprecipitate.** 10-20 mL/bag; contains 100 units factor VIII-C, 100 units factor vWF, 60 units factor XIII, and 250 mg fibrinogen; used for factor VIII deficiency and hemophilia A.
    - **F. Albumisol.** 5% and 25% (heat treated at 60 degrees C for 10 hrs).
- **III. Complications**
    - **A. Immune/non-hemolytic**
        1. **Febrile.** Most common (0.5-4.0% of transfusions); due to recipient antibodies against donor WBCs and platelets; treat with slow infusion and antipyretics.
        2. **Allergic.** Occurs in about 3% of transfusions; caused by immunoglobulin alloantibodies against substances in the donor plasma with activation of mast cells and histamine release; most commonly present with abrupt onset of pruritic erythema or urticaria on arms and trunk; treat with slow infusion and antihistamines.
        3. **Anaphylaxis.** Occurs in IgA deficient patients who have developed an

anti-IgA; immune complex activates mast cells, basophils, etc. resulting in hypotension, dyspnea, laryngeal edema, wheezing and possibly shock; treat like severe allergic reaction.

B. Immune/hemolytic

1. **Acute hemolytic transfusion reaction** occurs in 1:10,000 with 20-60% mortality; usually due to donor blood ABO incompatibility; complement activation leads to hemolysis and may result in DIC; clinically presents with headache, chills, nausea, vomiting, fever, flank pain, hypotension, dyspnea, bleeding and hemoglobinuria; acute renal failure may occur.
2. **Delayed hemolytic transfusion reaction:** occurs 1:2500; usually seen in previously sensitized patients.

C. Non-immune

1. Infections
   a. **AIDS.** Overall risk about 1:225,000 per unit.
   b. **Hepatitis B.** Risk is currently 1:200,000 per unit; accounts for 2% of transfusion related hepatitis.
   c. **Hepatitis C.** Risk is currently 1:3300 per unit; accounts for 98% of transfusion related hepatitis.
   d. **HTLV 1 and 2.** 4% chance of developing T-cell leukemia or spastic paraparesis; 1:50,000 per unit.
2. Metabolic
   a. Decreased pH. Reflecting lactate production.
   b. Increase potassium. Due to cell lysis; increases with length of storage.
   c. Decreased plasma bicarbonate.
   d. Increased PCO2.
   e. Decrease in 2,3 DPG: consumed by RBC's; P_{50} decreases to 18 mmHg after 1 week and 15 mmHg after 3 weeks.
3. Coagulopathy
   a. Usually occurs only after massive transfusion (greater than 10 units).
   b. Dilutional thrombocytopenia. Most common cause of abnormal bleeding in massive transfusion, responds quickly to platelet transfusions.
   c. Low Factors V and VIII. Factors V and VII are very labile in stored blood and may decrease to levels as low as 15-20% normal, however, this is usually enough for hemostasis.
   d. DIC. DIC is a hypercoaguable state caused by activation of the clotting system leading to deposition of fibrin in microvasculature which causes a secondary activation of fibrinolysis. results in consumption of factors and platelets.

IV. Massive transfusions

A. **Massive transfusion** is defined as the replacement of a patient's total blood volume in less than 24 hours, or as the acute administration of more than half the patient's estimated blood volume per hour.

B. **The use of universal donor blood** (group O, Rh negative blood)
1. Group O, Rh negative blood should be reserved for patients close to exsanguination. If time permits, cross-matched or uncross-matched type specific blood should be administered.
2. Group O, Rh negative blood should not be given as whole blood. The serum contains high anti-A and anti-B titers which may cause hemolysis of recipient red cells.

3. If more than 4 units of group O, Rh negative whole blood is administered, type-specific blood should not be given subsequently since the potentially high anti-A and anti-B titers could cause hemolysis of the donor blood.
4. Patients administered up to 10 units of group O, Rh negative packed red blood cells may be switched to type-specific blood, since there is an insignificant risk of hemolysis from the small volume of plasma administered with packed red blood cells.

C. Complications of massive transfusions

1. **Hypothermia.** Every effort should be made to use blood warmers. All blood products should be given through the blood warmer except platelets and cryoprecipitate.
2. **Impaired oxygen release** from hemoglobin. erythrocytic levels of 2,3-DPG decrease with stored blood.
3. **Coagulopathy**
   a. Dilutional thrombocytopenia is the most frequent bleeding disorder seen in trauma patients, but it rarely becomes a problem until at least 150-200% of the patient's blood volume has been replaced. However, thrombocytopenia can occur following smaller transfusions if disseminated intravascular coagulation (DIC) occurs or if there is pre-existing thrombocytopenia.
   b. Platelet activity in stored blood is only 5-10% of normal after 24-48 hours of storage.
   c. Most coagulation factors are stable in stored blood, except factors V and VII.
4. **Electrolytes and acid base abnormalities**
   a. Hyperkalemia or hypokalemia can occur with massive transfusion.
   b. The plasma potassium concentration of stored blood increases during storage and may be over 30 mmol/L. Hyperkalemia is generally not a problem unless very large amounts of blood are given quickly. Hypokalemia is more common as red cells begin active metabolism and intracellular uptake of potassium restarts.
   c. Acid-base status should be followed with blood gases. Lactic acid levels in the blood pack give stored blood an acid load of up to 30-40mmol/L.
5. **Citrate toxicity**
   a. Citrate intoxication is due to acutely decreased serum ionized calcium, because citrate chelates calcium.
   b. Empiric administration of calcium is not warranted unless ionized calcium is low.
   c. Each unit of blood contains approximately 3 g citrate, which binds ionized calcium. Transfusion at rates higher than one unit every five minutes or impaired liver function may result in citrate toxicity and hypocalcemia.
6. **Infection**
   a. HIV. 1:250,00 donor unit exposures.
   b. Post-transfusion hepatitis constitutes the principal viral risk of blood transfusion (incidence of 4-15%).

V. Alternatives to homologous blood transfusion
A. Autologous transfusion.
B. Donor-directed transfusion.
C. Perioperative blood salvage (cell saver).
D. Intraoperative isovolemic hemodilution.

Blood Therapy Management 101

E. Substitute products for replacement of plasma and blood volume.

VI. Coagulation tests

A. Partial thromboplastin time (PTT)
1. Partial thromboplastin is substituted for platelet phospholipid and eliminates platelet variability.
2. PTT measures the clotting ability of all factors in the intrinsic and common pathways except factor XIII.
3. PTT is abnormal if there are decreased amounts of coagulation factors, patients on heparin, or if there is a circulating anticoagulant present.
4. Normal values are between 25 and 37 seconds.

B. Activated partial thromboplastin time (aPTT)
1. An activator is added to the test tube before addition of partial thromboplastin added.
2. Maximal activation of the contact factors (XII and XI) eliminates the lengthy natural contact activation phase and results in more consistent and reproducible results.
3. Normal aPTT is 25-35 seconds.

C. Prothrombin time (PT)
1. Performed by measuring the time needed to form a clot when calcium and a tissue extract are added to plasma.
2. PT evaluates the activity of fibrinogen, prothrombin and factors V, VII and X.
3. Normal PT is 10-12 seconds (depending on control).

D. International normalized ratio (INR)
1. Developed to improve the consistency of oral anticoagulant therapy.
2. Converts the PT ratio to a value that would have been obtained using a standard PT method.
3. INR is calculated as $(Pt_{patient}/Pt_{normal})^{ISI}$ (ISI is the international sensitivity index assigned to the test system).

E. Thromboelastrogram
1. **Thromboelastography (TEG)** is a method of testing for global assessment of coagulation. This technique uses a small sample of blood placed in a slowly rotating cuvette at 37°C. A piston is suspended in the cuvette, and as the coagulation proceeds, the tension on the piston is measured. A tracing is generated and several parameters are measured (see below).
2. **Thromboelastrogram parameters**
   a. **r (reaction time).** start of recording until 1 mm deflection (represents initial fibrin formation).
   b. **k (clot formation time).** measured from r until there is a 20 mm deflection in the tracing.
   c. **a (angle).** slope of the increase from r time to k time.
   d. **MA.** maximum amplitude in millimeters, a measure of the maximum clot strength (dependent on fibrinogen, level, platelet numbers, and function).
   e. **A^{60}.** deflection measure at 60 minutes after MA (represents clot lysis and retraction).
3. **Sonoclot**. The Sonoclot is a test of whole blood that utilizes a warmed cuvette and a suspended piston apparatus, This piston vibrates up and down very rapidly in the blood sample and Sonoclot detects any impedance to this vibration. As a result, the test follows the changes

in viscosity over time.
4. **Activated clotting time (ACT).** The ACT provides a global measurement of hemostatic function and is measured after whole blood is exposed to a specific activator of coagulation. The time for in vitro clot formation after whole blood is exposed to diatomaceous earth (Celite) is defined as the ACT. Normal is 90 to 120 seconds. The linear increase in ACT seen with increasing doses of heparin provides a convenient method to monitor heparin's anticoagulant effect. Although the ACT test is simple, it lacks sensitivity to clotting abnormalities.

VII. Treatment of hemolytic transfusion reactions

A. **Stop the transfusion**

B. Maintain the urine output at a minimum of 75 to 100 ml/hr by the following methods. Generously administer fluids IV and possibly mannitol, 12.5 to 50 grams, given over a 5-15 minute period.

C. If IV administered fluids and mannitol are ineffective, than administer furosemide, 20-40 mg IV.

D. Alkalinize the urine since bicarbonate is preferentially excreted in the urine, only 40-70 mEq/70 kg of sodium bicarbonate is usually required to raise the urine pH to 8, whereupon repeat urine pH determinations indicate the need for additional bicarbonate.

E. Assay urine and plasma hemoglobin concentrations. Determine platelet count, PTT, serum fibrinogen level.

F. Return unused blood to blood bank for crossmatch and send blood sample for antibody screen and direct antiglobulin test. Prevent hypotension to ensure adequate renal blood flow.

VIII. Sickle Cell Anemia

A. Sickle cell anemia is a hemoglobinopathy that results from inheritance of a gene for a structurally abnormal beta globin chain. This results in HbS which has two forms.

B. **Sickle cell trait (HbAS)** is a heterozygous state. Only 1% of the red cells in heterozygote's venous circulation are sickled. These patients are usually asymptomatic. Vigorous physical activity at high altitude, air travel in unpressurized planes, and anesthesia are potentially hazardous.

C. **Sickle cell disease (HbSS).** homozygous state: 70-98% HbS.

D. **Clinical features**
1. Signs and symptoms include anemia (HgB levels 6.5 to 10 gm/dl), obstructive or hemolytic jaundice, joint and bone pain, abdominal and chest pains, lymphadenopathy, chronic leg ulcers, hematuria, epistaxis, priapism, finger clubbing, and skeletal deformities.
2. The disease is characterized by periodic exaggeration of symptoms or sickle cell crisis. There are four main types of crises.
    a. **Vaso-occlusive crises.** caused by sickled cells blocking the microvasculature, characterized by sudden onset of pain frequently with no clear-cut precipitating event.
    b. **Hemolytic crises.** seen in patients with sickle cell disease plus G-PD deficiency, has hematologic features of sudden hemolysis.
    c. **Sequestration crises.** involves sequestration of red blood cells in the liver and spleen causing their massive, sudden enlargement and an acute fall in peripheral hematocrit, this can progress to circulatory collapse.
    d. **Aplastic crises.** characterized by transient episodes of bone marrow depression commonly occurring after viral infection.

3. Anesthetic management
  a. The practice of transfusing these patients to an end point of having 70% hemoglobin A and less than 30% hemoglobin S cells before major surgery remains controversial.
  b. To lessen the risk of intraoperative sickling patients should be kept well oxygenated and well hydrated. Acidosis and hypothermia should also be avoided.

IX. Factor VIII deficiency (hemophilia A)
  A. The half life of factor VIII in plasma is 8-12 hours.
  B. Treatment consists of lyophilized factor VIII, cryoprecipitate, or desmopressin. Infusion of 1 unit of factor VIII per kg of body weight will increase the factor VIII activity level by 2%. Activity levels of 20-40% are recommended before surgery.
  C. Bleeding episodes are related to the level of factor VIII activity (normal activity is 100%).

X. Factor IX deficiency (hemophilia B; Christmas disease)
  A. The half life of factor IX in plasma is 24 hours.
  B. Therapy consists of factor IX concentrates of FFP. For surgical hemostasis, activity levels of 50% to 80% are necessary.
  C. Infusion of 1 unit of factor IX per kg of body weight will increase the factor IX activity level by 1%.

Spinal and Epidural Anesthesia

I. Contraindications to peridural anesthesia
A. Absolute contraindications
1. Lack of patient consent.
2. Localized infection at injection site.
3. Generalized sepsis or bacteremia.
4. Allergy to local anesthetics.
5. Increased intracranial pressure.
6. Coagulopathy

B. Relative contraindications
1. Localized infection peripheral to regional site.
2. Demyelinating central nervous system disease.
3. Chronic back pain or prior lumbar spine surgery.
4. Hypovolemia.
5. Patients taking platelet inhibiting drugs.

II. Spinal anesthesia (local anesthetic placed in the subarachnoid space)
A. Anatomy
1. **Spinal canal.** Extends from the foramen magnum to the sacral hiatus.
2. **Spinal cord.** Spinal cord extends the length of the vertebral canal during fetal life, ends at L3 at birth, and moves progressively cephalad to reach the adult position of L1-L2 by 2 years of age.
3. **Subarachnoid space.** Subarachnoid space lies between the pia mater and the arachnoid and extends from S2 to the cerebral ventricles.
4. **Course of anatomy to the subarachnoid space.** Skin, subcutaneous tissue, supraspinous ligament, interspinous ligament, ligamentum flavum, epidural space, and dura.

B. Physiological changes with spinal and epidural anesthesia
1. **Neural blockade**
   a. **Sequence of neural blockade**
      (1) Sympathetic block with peripheral vasodilation and skin temperature elevation.
      (2) Loss of pain and temperature sensation.
      (3) Loss of proprioception.
      (4) Loss of touch and pressure sensation.
      (5) Motor paralysis.
   b. The above sequence of neural blockade occurs because smaller C fibers are blocked more easily than the larger sensory fiber, which in turn are blocked more easily than motor fibers. As a result, the level of autonomic blockade extends above the level of the sensory blockade by 2-3 segments, while the motor blockade is 2-3 segments below the sensory blockade.
   c. With epidural anesthesia, the local anesthetics act directly on the spinal nerve roots located in the lateral part of the space. As a result, the onset of the block is slower than with spinal anesthesia, and the intensity of the sensory and motor block is less.

2. **Cardiovascular**
   a. **Hypotension.** The degree of hypotension is directly proportional to the degree of sympathetic blockade.
   b. **Blockade above T4** interrupts cardiac sympathetic fibers, leading to bradycardia, decreased cardiac output, and further decrease in

blood pressure.
3. **Respiratory.** With ascending height of the block into the thoracic area, there is a progressive, ascending intercostal muscle paralysis. The diaphragmatic ventilation is mediated by the phrenic nerve, and typically will remain unaffected even during high cervical blockade.
4. **Visceral effects**
   a. **Bladder.** Sacral blockade results in an atonic bladder.
   b. **Intestine.** With sympathectomy, vagal tone dominates and results in a small, contracted gut with active peristalsis.

III. Factors influencing spinal anesthetic
A. Dosage.
B. Drug volume.
C. Addition of vasoconstrictors (decrease vascular uptake and prolong action).
D. Baricity of the local anesthetic solution (specific gravity).
E. Shape of the spinal canal (when supine, a high point at L3-L4 and low point at T5-T6.
F. Position of the patient.
G. Intra-abdominal pressure. Increased intra-abdominal pressure, as seen with pregnancy, obesity, ascites, or abdominal tumors, increases the blood flow through the epidural venous plexus, reducing the volume of CSF, thus causing the local anesthetic to spread further.
H. Age (spinal space thought to become smaller with age).

IV. Complications of spinal anesthesia
A. **Hypotension.** Prehydrating with 500-1000 cc of crystalloid before performing the block will help decrease the incidence of hypotension.
B. **Paresthesia or nerve injury.** During placement of the needle or injection of anesthetic, direct trauma to a spinal nerve or intraneural injection may occur.
C. **Blood tap or vascular injury.** Needle may puncture an epidural vein during needle insertion.
D. **Nausea and vomiting.** Usually the result of hypotension or unopposed vagal stimulation.
E. **High spinal.** May see apnea with total spinal from direct blockade of C3-C5.
F. **Pain on injection.**
G. **Backache.** Overall the incidence of backache following spinal anesthesia is no different from that following general anesthesia.
H. **Postdural puncture headache.** Usually seen 6-48 hours after dural puncture (see below).
I. **Urinary retention.** Urinary retention may outlast the sensory and motor blockade.
J. **Infection.** Meningitis, arachnoiditis, and epidural abscess may occur, but are exceedingly rare.

V. Factors influencing epidural anesthesia
A. Local anesthetic selected.
B. Mass of drug injected (dose, volume, and concentration).
C. Addition of vasoconstrictors (epinephrine) to reduce systemic absorption.
D. Site injection.
E. Patients over 40 years of age.
F. Pregnancy (hormonal and/or mechanical factors).

106 Spinal and Epidural Anesthesia

VI. Complications of epidural anesthesia
   A. Dural puncture. Unintentional dural puncture occurs in 1% of epidural injections performed.

   B. Catheter complications
   1. Inability to insert the catheter.
   2. Catheter can be inserted into an epidural vein.
   3. Catheters can break off or become knotted within the epidural space.

   C. Unintentional subarachnoid injection.

   D. Intravascular injection. May result in local anesthetic overdose where large amounts of local anesthetic are used.

   E. Direct spinal cord injury. Possible if the injection is above L2 in the adult patient.

   F. Bloody tap. May result from perforation of an epidural vein.

VII. Postdural puncture headache
   A. Characteristics of a postdural puncture headache
   1. Postural component (made worse by upright position).
   2. Frontal or occipital location.
   3. Tinnitus.
   4. Diplopia.
   5. Young females.
   6. Use of a large-gauge needle.

   B. Mechanism
   1. Usually due to a continued leak of CSF through the hole in the dura mater, resulting in low CSF pressure, which causes traction on meningeal vessels and nerves.
   2. Incidence. the overall incidence is approximately 5-10%.

   C. Treatment of a postdural puncture headache
   1. Oral Analgesics.
   2. Bed rest.
   3. Hydration (IVF, PO fluids, caffeine containing beverages).
   4. Caffeine infusion (500 mg caffeine and sodium benzoate in 1 liter of isotonic crystalloid given over 1-2 hours).
   5. Epidural blood patch (placement of 10-20 cc of autologous blood in the epidural space). The success rate is approximately 95%.

Neuraxial Opioids: Side effects and treatment		
Problem	**Treatment Options**	**Notes**
Pruritus	Nalbuphine 5-10 mg IV/IM Diphenhydramine 25-50 mg IV Naloxone 40-80 mcg IV	May be severe after intrathecal morphine
Nausea/Vomiting	Metoclopramide 5-10 mg IV Nalbuphine 5-10 mg IV/IM Naloxone 40-80 mcg IV	
Respiratory Depression	Naloxone 0.1 mg IV prn	Watch for synergism with other sedatives
Urinary Retention	Urinary Catheter	

Problem	Treatment Options	Notes
Blood Pressure Changes	Fluid hydration Ephedrine Phenylephrine	Most likely after meperidine (local anesthetic effects)

Regional Anesthesia

I. General information
  A. Paresthesia
   1. Placing a needle in direct contact with a nerve or within the substance of the nerve will stimulate that nerve causing paraesthesias.
   2. Injection into a perineural location often results in a brief accentuation of the paraesthesia; in contrast, an intraneural injection produces an intense, searing pain that signals the need to immediately terminate the injection.
   3. Correct needle placement can be determined by elicitation of paraesthesia, perivascular sheath technique, transarterial placement, and a nerve stimulator.

  B. Regional block needles
   1. **Blunt-bevel needle.** Designed to minimize trauma upon direct contact with nerves. The angle of the bevel is increased 20-30 degrees, and the sharpness is decreased.
   2. **Insulated needle.** A nonconductor is bonded to the needle except for the last millimeter before the bevel.
   3. **The beaded needle.** A regional needle designed for use with a nerve stimulator.

II. Brachial plexus block
  A. Interscalene block
   1. **Technique.** The needle is inserted in the interscalene groove at the level of the cricoid cartilage and advanced perpendicular to the skin until a paresthesia is elicited or a transverse spinous process is contacted, at which point 30-40 cc of local anesthetic is injected.
   2. **Indications.** Any procedure on the upper extremity, including the shoulder. This technique has a high rate of failure to achieve full block of the ulnar nerve (10-20%) for hand surgery.
   3. **Special contraindications.** Contralateral phrenic paresis, severe asthma.
   4. **Side effects.** Horner's syndrome, phrenic paresis.
   5. **Complications.** Proximity of the vertebral artery makes intraarterial injection possible with rapid progression to grand mal seizure after small amounts are injected. The neural foramina can be reached, and massive epidural, subarachnoid, or subdural injection can occur. Stellate ganglion block results in Horner's sign (myosis, ptosis, anhidrosis). Other complications include recurrent laryngeal nerve block (30-50%) leading to hoarseness, phrenic nerve block, pneumothorax, infection, bleeding, and nerve injury.

  B. Supraclavicular block
   1. **Indications.** Operations on the upper arm, elbow, lower arm and hand.
   2. **Special contraindications.** Hemorrhagic diathesis, contralateral

phrenic paresis.
    3. **Side effects.** Horner's syndrome, phrenic paresis.
    4. **Complications.** Pneumothorax (1-6%) and hemothorax are the most common. Phrenic nerve block and Horner's syndrome may occur.
  C. **Axillary block**
    1. **Indications.** Operations on the lower arm and hand.
    2. **Anatomy.** It should be noted that in the axilla, the musculocutaneous nerve has already left its sheath and lies within the coracobrachialis.
    3. **Special contraindications.** Lymphangitis (presumed infected axillary nodes).
    4. **Complications.** Puncture of the axillary artery, intravenous/intra-arterial injection (systemic toxic reaction), postoperative neuropathies (more common when multiple sites of paresthesia are elicited).
III. **Techniques of identifying placement of the needle**
  A. **Fascial "clicks".** Feel a "click" as the needle advances and penetrates the sheath.
  B. **Paresthesia technique.** Patient cooperation is essential. Instruct the patient to say "stop" if and when they experience paresthesia.
IV. **Regional Anesthesia in Pediatrics**
  A. **Pharmacology**
    1. Protein binding of local anesthetics is decreased in neonates because of decreased of albumin.
    2. Increased volume of distribution may decrease free local anesthetic concentrations.
  B. **Spinal anesthesia**
    1. Usually performed in sitting position.
    2. A 22-gauge, 1.5 inch spinal needle is commonly used in infants. In children older than 2 years a 25-26 gauge needle can be used.
    3. **Hypobaric solutions** are most commonly used.
      a. **Bupivacaine** 0.75% in 8.25% dextrose, 0.3 mg/kg in infants and children.
      b. **Tetracaine** 1% with equal volume 10% dextrose, 0.8-1.0 mg/kg in infants and 0.25-0.5 mg/kg in children.
      c. **Duration** may be prolonged with the addition of epinephrine 10 mcg/kg (up to 0.2 mg).
    4. **Complications**
      a. Anesthetic level recedes faster in children than adults.
      b. Hypotension is rare in children under 10 years.
      c. Contraindicated in children with CNS anatomic defects and a history of grade III-IV intraventricular hemorrhage.
  C. **Caudal and lumbar epidural anesthesia**
    1. Dural sac in the neonate ends at S3.
    2. **Caudal catheters**
      a. **Infants.** 22 g catheter placed (40-50 mm) through 20 g Tuohy needle.
      b. **Children.** 20 g catheter placed (90-100 mm) through 17-18 g Tuohy needle.
    3. **Epidural catheters.** In older children use 20 g catheter with 18 g Touhy needle.
    4. **Drugs**
      a. **Single dose.** Bupivacaine 0.125% -0.25% with epinephrine. 1.5-2.5 mg/kg or 0.06 cc local anesthetic/kg/segment (segments are

counted from S5).
- **b. Intermittent bolus.** 1% lidocaine, 0.5 cc/kg followed by 0.5% lidocaine, 0.5 cc/kg every hour as needed.
- **c. Continuous infusion**
  - **(1)** Infants and children less than 7 years: load with 0.04 cc/kg/segment of 0.1% bupivacaine (with or without fentanyl 2-3 mcg/cc).
  - **(2)** Children older than 7 years load with 0.02 cc/kg/segment of 0.1% bupivacaine (with or without fentanyl 2-3 mcg/cc).
  - **(3)** Infusions of 0.1% bupivacaine (with or without fentanyl 2-3 mcg/cc) at 0.1 cc/kg/hr. May be increased up to 0.3 cc/kg/hr.
  - **(4)** Fentanyl should not be used in infants under 1 year.

Pediatric Anesthesia

Basic Pediatric Anesthesia Drugs

Atracurium	0.5 mg/kg	Meperidine (IM)	1 mg/kg
Atropine	0.01-0.02 mg/kg	STP (IV)	4-6 mg/kg
Fentanyl	3-5 mcg/kg	STP (PR)	25-30 mg/kg
Glycopyrrolate	5-10 mcg/kg	Succinylcholine	1-1.5 mg/kg
Neostigmine	0.05 mg/kg	Vecuronium	0.1 mg/kg
Chloral Hydrate	50-100 mg/kg	Versed (IV)	0.07-0.08 mg/kg
Diazepam (IV)	0.1 mg/kg	Methohexital (IV)	1-2 mg/kg
Droperidol	0.01-0.05 mg/kg	Morphine	0.05-0.1 mg/kg
Ephedrine	0.1 mg/kg	Naloxone	0.1 mg/kg
Furosemide	0.2-1 mg/kg	Pentobarbital (IM)	4-6 mg/kg
Ketamine (IV)	1-2 mg/kg	Tylenol	10-15 mg/kg
Ketamine (IM)	5-10 mg/kg	Versed (nasal)	0.3 mg/kg
Meperidine (IV)	0.02-2.0 mg/kg	Versed (PO)	0.5-1.0 mg/kg

Pediatric Emergency Drugs

Epinephrine	0.01-0.02 mg/kg	Epinephrine	0.1-1.0 mcg/kg/min
Verapamil	0.1-0.3 mg/kg	Dopamine	2-20 mcg/kg/min
Na Bicarbonate	0.5-2 mEq/kg	Dobutamine	5-20 mcg/kg/min
peds 8.4%:	1 mEq/cc	Isoproterenol	0.1-1.0 mcg/kg/min
neonatal 4.2%:	0.5 mEq/cc	Nitroprusside	0.5-8 mcg/kg/min
Calcium Cl	10-30 mg/kg	Lidocaine	20-50 mcg/kg/min
Ca Gluconate	30-60 mg/kg	Norepinephrine	0.1-1 mcg/kg/min
Lidocaine	1 mg/kg	Digoxin	0.02-0.04 mg/kg
Bretylium	5-10 mg/kg	Defibrillation	2-4 J/kg
Glucose (D25%)	0.5-1.0 gm/kg	Cardioversion	0.25-0.5 J/kg

Pediatric Airway Management

Pediatric Endotracheal Tube Sizes And Laryngoscope Blade Size		
Age	Size	Blade
Under 1500 gm	2.5	Miller 0: neonate/premature
1500-5000 gm	3.0	Miller 1: up to 6 - 8 months
Infant	3.0 - 3.5	Wis-Hipple 1.5: 9 months- 2 yrs
6 - 12 months	3.5 - 4.0	Miller 2: 2.5 - 5.0 years
12 - 20 months	4.0	Macintosh 2: child over 5 yrs
Over 20 months	4.0 + Age (yrs)/4	

Pediatric Endotracheal Tube Recommendations

I. **Endotracheal Tube Leak:** 15-20 cm H_2O.
II. **Length of Insertion of ETT**
   1. Under 1 year: 6 + Wt(kg).
   2. Over 1 year: 12 + Age/2.
   3. Add 2-3 cm for nasal tube.
III. **Uncuffed ETT** generally used for patients under 10 yrs.

Pediatric Vital Signs				
Age	RR	HR	SBP	DBP
Preterm	60	120-180	45-60	30
Neonate	40	100-180	55-70	40
12 months	30	100-140	70-100	60
3 years	25	85-115	75-110	70
5-12 years	20	80-100	80-120	70

Age And Approximate Weight
28 weeks = 1 kg +/- 100 g/wk from 22-30 weeks
<1 year: ½ age (months) plus 4 kg
1 yr to puberty: 2 times age in yrs plus 10 kg

112 Pediatric Anesthesia

I. Physiologic Differences (as compared to an adult)
   A. Cardiac. Cardiac output of neonates and infants is dependent on heart rate, since stroke volume is relatively fixed by a noncompliant and poorly developed left ventricle. The sympathetic nervous system and baroreceptor reflexes are not fully mature. The hallmark of hypovolemia is hypotension without tachycardia.
   B. Respiratory. Increased respiratory rate; tidal volume and dead space per kg are constant; lower functional residual capacity; lower lung compliance; greater chest wall compliance. Small alveoli are associated with low lung compliance. Hypoxic and hypercapnic ventilatory drives are not well developed in neonates and infants. Neonates are obligate nose breathers.
   C. Metabolism/temperature. Higher ratio of body surface area to body weight; heat production in neonates is nonshivering thermogenesis by metabolism of brown fat.
   D. Renal. Normal renal function by 6 months of age; premature neonates may posses decreased creatinine clearance, impaired sodium retention, glucose excretion, and bicarbonate reabsorption. Hypoglycemia is defined as <30 mg/dL in the neonate, and <40 mg/dL in older children.

II. Anatomical Differences--Airway. Larger head and tongue, narrow nasal passages, cephalad (and anterior appearing) larynx (opposite C4 versus C6 in adults), long omega-shaped epiglottis, short trachea and neck; cricoid cartilage narrowest point of airway in children younger than 5 years of age (glottis in adults).

III. Pharmacologic Differences
   A. Pediatric drug dosing is based upon a per-kilogram recommendation.
   B. Inhalational anesthetics. Higher alveolar ventilation, relatively low functional residual capacity (ie, a higher ratio of minute ventilation to functional residual capacity) contribute to a rapid rise in alveolar anesthetic concentration. The blood/gas coefficients of isoflurane and halothane are lower in neonates than adults. The minimum alveolar concentration is higher in infants than in neonates or adults. The blood pressure of neonates and infants tends to be more sensitive to volatile anesthetics.
   C. Nonvolatile anesthetics. Some barbiturates and opiate agonist appear to be more toxic in neonates than adults.
   D. Muscle relaxants. Infants require higher doses of succinylcholine per kilogram than do adults because of their larger volume of distribution. Children are more subject to cardiac dysrhythmias, myoglobinemia, hyperkalemia, and MH after succinylcholine than adults.

IV. Anesthetic Considerations for Specific Pediatric Disorders
   A. Prematurity. Prematurity is defined as birth before 37 weeks gestation or weight less than 2500 grams; premature infants are at increased risk for retinopathy of prematurity and apnea of prematurity.
   B. Apnea of prematurity. Factors that increase the risks of postoperative apnea and bradycardia are postconceptual age less than 52 weeks, necrotizing enterocolitis, neurologic problems and anemia. Regional anesthesia may be associated with a lower incidence. Usually occurs in the first 12 hours postoperatively. Patients should be monitored for 12-24 hours postoperatively. Caffeine (5-10 mg IV) decreases the incidence. Theophylline also effective.
   C. Congenital diaphragmatic hernia. Three types (left or right posterolateral foramen of Bochdalek or anterior foramen of Morgagni)

with left most common; a reduction in alveoli and bronchioli (pulmonary hypolpasia) is accompanied by marked elevation in pulmonary vascular resistance; hallmarks include hypoxia, scaphoid abdomen, bowel in the thorax; gastric distention should be minimized by placement of a nasogastric tube and avoidance of high levels of positive-pressure ventilation; sudden fall in lung compliance, blood pressure or oxygenation may signal a contralateral pneumothorax. Hyperventilation is recommended to decrease PVR and minimize right-to-left shunting.

D. **Tracheoesophageal fistula.** Most common is combination of upper esophagus that ends in a blind pouch and a lower esophagus that connects to the trachea; breathing results in gastric distention; intubate awake without muscle relaxants. Aspiration pneumonia and the coexistence of other congenital anomalies are common. The key to successful management is correct endotracheal tube position (the tip of the tube should lie between the fistula and the carina).

E. **Hypertrophic pyloric stenosis.** Persistent vomiting depletes sodium, potassium, chloride, and hydrogen ions, causing hypochloremic metabolic alkalosis. Initially, the kidney compensate for the alkalosis by excreting sodium bicarbonate in the urine. Later, as hyponatemia and dehydration worsen, the kidneys must conserve sodium even at the expense of hydrogen ion excretion (resulting in paradoxic aciduria). Correction should be with sodium chloride supplemented with potassium. Electrolyte abnormalities must be corrected prior to surgery. Neonates may be at increased risk for respiratory depression and hypoventilation postoperatively because of persistent metabolic or CSF alkalosis.

F. **Gastroschisis.** Defect in abdominal wall (lateral to umbilicus); no hernial sac; no associated congenital anomalies. The neonate remains intubated after the procedure and is weaned from the ventilator over the next 1-2 days. Insure adequate muscle relaxation.

G. **Omphalocele.** Defect in abdominal wall at the base of the umbilicus; hernial sac present; associated with congenital anomalies (trisomy 21, cardiac anomalies, diaphragmatic hernia, bladder anomalies).

H. **Croup (laryngotracheobronchitis).** Subglottic obstruction; viral etiology (parainfluenza 3); gradual onset follows upper respiratory tract infection; low grade fever; minimal drooling; normal WBC; biphasic stridor; retractions; hoarseness; barking cough; age 3 months to 3 years; rarely requires intubation.

I. **Acute epiglottis.** Bacterial infection (Hemophilus influenza type B); most commonly in 2 to 6 year olds; progresses rapidly from a sore throat to dysphagia and complete supraglottic airway obstruction; drooling; high fever; high WBC; treat with antibiotics and intubation (laryngoscopy should not be performed before induction of anesthesia because of possibility of laryngospasm).

J. **Necrotizing enterocolitis.** Acquired intestinal tract necrosis that appears in the absence of functional or anatomic lesions. Predominantly in premature. Systemic signs include temperature instability, lethargy, respiratory and circulatory instability, oliguria, and bleeding diathesis. Avoid nitrous oxide.

Cardiac Surgery

Pediatric Cardiovascular Physiology

I. **Fetal circulation**
   A. Acidosis, sepsis, hypothermia, hypoxia, and hypercarbia may cause reopening of the fetal shunts and persistence of the fetal circulation.
   B. Diagnosis of persistent pulmonary hypertension of the newborn can be confirmed by measurement of the PaO_2 in blood obtained simultaneously from preductal (right radial) and postductal (umbilical, posterior tibial, dorsalis pedis) arteries. A difference of 20 mmHg verifies the diagnosis.

II. **Closure of the ductus arteriosus**
   A. In the fetus, patency of the ductus arteriosus is maintained by high levels of prostaglandin (PGI_2 and PGE_1).
   B. Functional closure occurs by contraction of the smooth muscle of the ductal wall and usually occurs 10-15 hours after birth. An increase in PO_2 and a decrease in prostaglandins at birth contribute to functional closure.
   C. Permanent anatomic closure of the duct occurs in 4 to 6 weeks.

III. **Closure of the foramen ovale**
   A. Increase in left atrial over right atrial pressure functionally closes the foramen ovale.
   B. Anatomic closure of the foramen ovale occurs between 3 months and 1 year of age, although 20%-30% of adults and 50% of children less than 5 years of age have a probe-patent foramen ovale.

IV. **Closure of the ductus venosus**
   A. Decrease in umbilical venous blood flow causes passive closure of the ductus venosus.
   B. The ductus venosus is functionally closed by 1 week of life and anatomically closed by 3 weeks.

Cardiac Surgery

I. **Premedication for adult patients**
   A. Common premedications for cardiac surgery include morphine 0.1-0.15 mg/kg IM, scopolamine 0.3-0.4 mg IM, diazepam 0.15 mg/kg or lorazepam 0.06 mg/kg PO approximately 1-2 hours prior to surgery. The dose of scopolamine should be reduced to 0.2 mg for patients older than 70 years of age.
   B. The dose of premedication should be reduced in patients with critical aortic or mitral stenosis, those undergoing cardiac transplantation, patients with CHF, and patients with renal or hepatic dysfunction.
   C. Patients on heparin should not receive any IM medications. A common predication for heparinized patients includes diazepam 0.15 mg/kg PO (or lorazepam 0.04 mg/kg) and morphine 1-10 mg IV.
   D. Premedications should be given approximately 1-2 hours prior to the patient coming down to the operating room.

Valvular Heart Disease

Disease	Heart Rate	Rhythm	Preload	Afterload	Contractility	Blood Pressure
Aortic Stenosis	normal (70-80) avoid tachycardia	sinus is essential	increase or maintain	maintain	maintain	maintain
Aortic Regurgitation	normal or slight increase	sinus	maintain or increase	reduce	maintain or increase	maintain
Mitral Stenosis	normal (70-80) avoid tachycardia	sinus, A-fib ok, should digitalize	maintain or increase	maintain, avoid increased PVR	maintain	avoid hypotension
Mitral Regurgitation	normal or increase	usually A-fib, should digitalize	maintain	reduce	maintain or increase	maintain
Ischemic Heart Dz	slow rate	sinus	maintain	reduce	maintain or decrease	normal at rest
IHSS	normal or slight decrease	sinus, consider pacing	maintain or increase	maintain or slight increase	maintain or decrease	maintain

II. Premedications for pediatric patients

A. IM premedication
1. Under 6 months: atropine 10-20 mcg/kg IM (min 100 mcg).
2. 6-12 months: atropine 10-20 mcg/kg IM (min 100 mcg) plus morphine 0.10-0.15 mg/kg.
3. Over one year: atropine 10-20 mcg/kg IM (min 100 mcg) or scopolamine 0.015 mg/kg IM (max of 0.4 mg) or glycopyrrolate 0.004 mg/kg IM (max of 0.3 mg) plus morphine 0.1-0.2 mg/kg IM.

B. Oral premedication
1. Under 6 months: atropine 20 mcg/kg PO.
2. 6-12 months: pentobarbital 2-4 mg/kg PO +/- PO atropine.
3. Over one year: pentobarbital 2-4 mg/kg PO + Demerol 1-2 mg/kg PO (0.5-1.0 mg/kg Demerol in one year olds) +/- PO atropine.

III. Other orders and medications
A. Current cardiac medications should be continued; diuretics are usually held except in patients with CHF or afternoon cases.

B. Nasal canula oxygen (2-4 liters per minute) should be ordered along with the premedication (ie, oxygen should be given to all patients given premedications).

C. Patients undergoing rigid bronchoscopy or therapeutic bronchoscopy should receive an anticholinergic agent to minimize secretions (glycopyrrolate 0.2 mg IM).

IV. Intraoperative management for cardiac surgery

A. Prebypass period
1. This period is characterized by variable levels of stimulation. Stimulating periods include sternal splitting and retraction, pericardial incision, and aortic root dissection and cannulation.
2. Baseline laboratory data, including ABG, Hct, and ACT, should be obtained.

3. During sternal splitting, the lungs should be deflated.
4. Aortic root dissection and cannulation: this period can be very stimulating and should be treated aggressively with short-acting agents to minimize the risk of aortic tear or dissection.
5. **Heparinization**
   a. Heparin 300 IU/kg (400 IU/kg if receiving IV heparin). Administration is through a centrally placed catheter; aspirate blood both before and after injection.
   b. Check an ACT 5 minutes after heparin administration to monitor the degree of anticoagulation. ACT should be greater than 400 seconds prior to initiating cardiopulmonary bypass. If needed, an additional 100-200 IU/kg is administered.

B. Checklist prior to initiating cardiopulmonary bypass
1. Ensure adequate heparinization.
2. Turn nitrous oxide off.
3. Pulmonary artery catheter should be pulled back 3-5 cm.
4. Turn transesophageal echo off.

C. Bypass period
1. Once adequate flows and venous drainage are established, volatile anesthetics, IV fluids, and positive-pressure ventilation are discontinued.
2. Measure ACT to ensure adequate heparinization.
3. Frequent ABGs (uncorrected), hematocrit, potassium, calcium levels should be obtained.
4. Watch for the following complications
   a. **Hypotension**
      (1) Venous cannula. Kink, malposition, clamp, air lock.
      (2) Inadequate venous return. Bleeding hypovolemia, IVC obstruction.
      (3) Pump. Poor occlusion, low flows.
      (4) Arterial cannula. Misdirected, kinked, partially clamped, dissection.
      (5) Vasodilation. Anesthetics, hemodilution, idiopathic.
      (6) Transducer or monitoring malfunction, stopcocks the wrong way.
   b. **Hypertension**
      (1) Pump. Increased flow.
      (2) Arterial cannula. Misdirected.
      (3) Vasoconstriction. Light anesthesia, response to temperature changes.
      (4) Transducer or monitor malfunction.
      (5) Monitor patients' facial appearance. Suffusion (inadequate SVC drainage), unilateral blanching (innominate artery cannulation).
      (6) Check adequacy of perfusion by monitoring flow and pressure, acidosis, and mixed venous oxygen saturation.

D. Checklist prior to terminating cardiopulmonary bypass
1. Check labs. Hematocrit (22-25% is ideal), ABGs, potassium, glucose, and calcium.
2. Lungs ventilated with 100% oxygen.
3. Look at the heart to evaluate overall function.
4. Core temperature should be at least 37°C.

5. Stable rhythm (preferably sinus rhythm) with adequate heart rate (80-100 beats/min).
6. All monitors on and recalibrated.

E. Post-separation from cardiopulmonary bypass
1. Pressure maintenance. transfuse from CPB reservoir to maintain left atrial pressure or PA occlusion pressure. Optimal filling is determined by blood pressure, cardiac output, and direct observation of the heart.
2. Low cardiac output (despite adequate filling pressure and rhythm) may indicate the need for a positive inotrope. Dopamine is a first-line agent. Dobutamine and amrinone are alternatives.
3. High cardiac output but low blood pressure should be a vasoconstrictor.
4. Hypertension. Should be treated to prevent bleeding at the suture lines and cannulation sites.
5. RV dysfunction. Noted by CVP rising out of proportion to left atrial pressure. Treat with the following:
   a. Treat know causes of elevated PVR. light anesthesia, hypercarbia, hypoxemia, and acidemia.
   b. Vasodilator therapy. Nitroglycerin, nitroprusside or PGE1.
   c. Inotropic support.

F. Period after CPB
1. Hemodynamic stability is the primary goal.
2. Hemostasis. Once hemodynamic stability is achieved, protamine can be administered.
   a. Initially 25-50 mg is given over 5 minutes, and the hemodynamic response is observed.
   b. Monitor PA pressures while administering.
   c. In general, 1 mg of protamine is administered for each 1 mg of heparin given.
   d. After protamine administration, check ACT and compare to baseline. Additional protamine can be given if needed.
   e. During transfusion of heparinized pump blood, additional protamine (25-50 mg) should be given.

V. Acid-base management during CPB
A. pH-stat.
Requires temperature correction for interpretation of blood gases during CPB. Temperature correction can be accomplished by setting the blood gas analyzer to measure the patient's temperature. A pH of 7.40 and a $PaCO_2$ of 40 mmHg when the patient is cold requires the addition of CO_2.

B. Alpha-stat.
Requires no temperature correction for interpreting blood gases. The sample is warmed to 37 degrees C. and then measured in the blood gas analyzer as any other sample. The addition of CO_2 is usually not necessary.

VI. Post-cardiopulmonary bypass bleeding
A. Differential diagnosis
1. Uncorrected surgical defects.
2. Circulating anticoagulants. residual heparin and heparin rebound, protamine anticoagulation
3. Platelet defects. platelet function defect, thrombocytopenia.

B. Treatment
1. Circulating anticoagulants. adequate heparinization should be confirmed with ACT, and additional protamine given if needed.

2. Platelet abnormalities. usually given after other coagulation deficiencies have been corrected and no surgically correctable lesion exists.
3. Deficiencies of circulating procoagulants should be corrected by infusing FFP, cryoprecipitate, or fresh donor blood.

VII. Prevention
A. Pharmacological factors
1. **Desmopressin**
   a. Synthetic product that increases plasma levels of Factor VIII and Von Willebrand factor and decreases bleeding times.
   b. Dosing. 0.3 mcg/kg IV given over 20-30 min.
   c. Side effects. Decreased free water clearance from ADH activity, hypotension, thrombosis, decreased serum sodium, hyponatremic seizures.
2. **Aprotinin**. Inhibitor of several proteases and factor XIIa activation of complement (see selected drug section)
3. **Antifibrinolytic agents**
   a. Epsilon aminocaproic acid (Amicar)
      (1) Synthetic antifibrinolytics. Inhibits proteolytic activity of plasmin and conversion of plasminogen to plasmin by plasminogen activator.
      (2) Dose. Loading dose 100-150 mg/kg IV followed by constant infusion of 10-15 mg/kg/h.
   b. Tranexamic acid
      (1) Similar mechanism as epsilon aminocaproic acid but is approximately 10 times more potent.
      (2) Dose. Loading dose 10 mg/kg IV followed by infusion of 1 mg/kg/hr.
   c. Complications of antifibrinolytics
      (1) Bleeding into kidneys or ureters may thrombose and obstruct the upper urinary tract.
      (2) Contraindicated if DIC.
      (3) Hypotension may occur with rapid administration.
      (4) May be associated with thrombosis and subsequent stroke, myocardial infarction or deep vein thrombosis.

Automatic Implantable Cardioverter Defibrillator

I. Common indications for AICD implantation
A. Patients with a history of near-sudden death who have not responded to drug therapy and are not candidates for arrhythmia surgery.
B. Patients who have had unsuccessful arrhythmia surgery.
C. Post cardiac arrest patients who have not had an MI and who have no inducible arrhythmia during electrophysiologic testing.
D. Patients undergoing endocardial resection for recurrent VT.

II. Contraindications
A. Uncontrolled congestive heart failure.
B. Frequent recurrences of VT that would rapidly deplete the battery.

III. Surgical techniques
A. Nonthoracotomy approach. this approach employs either a single or multiple endocardial electrodes positioned fluoroscopically.
B. Thoracotomy approaches

Cardiac Surgery 119

1. Median sternotomy.
2. Left thoracotomy.
3. Subxiphoid approach.
4. Subcostal approach.

IV. Intraoperative testing

A. The purpose of intraoperative testing is to establish the defibrillation threshold (i.e., the minimum energy required to defibrillate the heart to a stable rhythm). Internal paddles should be readily available in the operative field during the entire procedure, and external patches should also be placed preoperatively.

B. The initial step is to ensure adequate sensing capability.

C. The leads are connected to an external cardioverter-defibrillator unit. This device can deliver programmable shocks of 1 to 40 J to defibrillate the heart.

D. Ventricular fibrillation is induced via rapid ventricular pacing or alternating current. A period of 10 to 20 seconds of fibrillation follows in order to ensure that spontaneous cardioversion will not occur.

E. The ECD unit is activated and discharged to determine the defibrillation threshold (the lowest amount of energy required to reliably attain a stable rhythm. Approximately 6 to 8 defibrillations are usually necessary to test the system. Amiodarone or hypokalemia may be responsible for high defibrillation thresholds.

F. If all the tests performed with the ECD unit are successful, an AICD is connected to the leads and ventricular fibrillation is again induced to test the newly implanted unit.

V. Anesthetic considerations

A. Preoperative assessment

1. A thorough preoperative evaluation should be preformed. The indication for the AICD should be noted.
2. Many patients will be taking antidysrhythmic agents at the time of surgery. In theory, the device and defibrillation thresholds should be tested while the patient is on the drug regimen that is planned postoperatively.
3. Antidysrhythmic agent of concern is amiodarone, which is negative inotropic agent and vasodilator. Amiodarone may cause refractory bradycardia or may precipitate a profound and prolonged hypotensive state postoperatively.

B. Intraoperatively monitoring.
Standard monitors and an arterial line are the minimum required monitors. Central venous access may be considered for administration of vasoactive drugs. Pulmonary catheter is depends on the patients cardiac status. Usually, however, a pulmonary artery catheter is not required for this procedure.

C. Anesthetic technique.
General anesthesia with nitrous oxide, narcotic, and muscle relaxant anesthetic is most common. This technique has minimal effects upon the induction of VT.

D. Other considerations

1. The cardioversion is commonly associated with transient hypertension and tachycardia, probably caused by sympathetic outflow.
2. Multiple intraoperative inductions of VT or VF may cause profound hypotension.
3. External defibrillator must be available.
4. Isoproterenol infusion occasionally has been administered to facilitate dysrhythmia induction.

5. The AICD is occasionally inactivated after being placed to avoid the cautery from trigger the AICD to discharge. The AICD is reactivated postoperatively.

E. AICD complications
1. Pacemaker interaction
   A. Both temporary and permanent pacemakers may interact with a AICD by interfering with dysrhythmia detection.
   B. The AICD can be deactivated when using temporary pacing, especially, A-V sequential pacing.
2. Mechanical. lead fractures, lead insulation breaks, and lead migration.
3. Rate miscounting leading to unnecessary shocks.
4. Infection.

Elective Cardioversion

I. Preoperative evaluation
A. Patients should NPO prior to the procedure.
B. 12 lead electrocardiogram should be preformed before the procedure to confirm that the arrhythmia is still present.
C. Preoperative labs should be within normal limits (metabolic and electrolyte disorders should be corrected).

II. Monitoring
A. Standard ASA monitors should be used.
B. Reliable intravenous access.
C. Other equipment should include an ambu bag, suction, airway supplies, anesthetic drugs, and crash cart.

III. Anesthetic technique
A. Premedication is not usually necessary.
B. A brief period of amnesia or a light general anesthetic is all that is usually required. This can be accomplished with etomidate, methohexital, propofol, or a benzodiazepine.
C. Following preoxygenation with 100% oxygen, the sedative-hypnotic is given. As soon as consciousness is lost, the appropriate charge may be delivered. The airway is maintained and ventilation is supported until consciousness is regained.

IV. Complications of cardioversion.
Transient myocardial depression, postshock arrhythmias, and arterial embolism.

Vascular Surgery

I. **Carotid artery surgery** (carotid endarterectomy; CEA)
   A. **Preoperative considerations**
      1. **Indications.** TIAs associated with ipsilateral severe carotid stenosis (>70% occlusion), severe ipsilateral stenosis in a patient with a minor (incomplete) stroke, and 30-70% occlusion in a patient with ipsilateral symptoms (usually an ulcerated plaque), emboli arising from a carotid lesion, large ulcerated plaque.
      2. **Operative mortality** is 1-4% and is primarily due to cardiac complications.
      3. **Perioperative morbidity** is 4-10%. Stroke is the most common and expected major complication during and after carotid endarterectomy. Hypertension occurs in about 70% of patients undergoing carotid endarterectomy and is associated with an increase in the risk of stroke.
      4. **Complications.** Hematoma with tracheal compression, supraglottic edema, cranial nerve injury (cranial nerves VII, IX, X, and XII), myocardial infarction, intraparenchymal hemorrhage, carotid occlusion, intracerebral hemorrhage, embolism.
   B. **Preoperative anesthetic evaluation.** Most patients undergoing CEA are elderly and hypertensive, with generalized arteriosclerosis. Preoperative evaluation should include a through cardiac and neurologic evaluation.
   C. **Anesthesia technique**
      1. The anesthesia goal is to maintain adequate cerebral perfusion without stressing the heart. In addition, the patient should be sufficiently responsive immediately after surgery to obey commands and thereby facilitate neurologic evaluation.
      2. Mean arterial blood pressure should be maintained at or slightly above the patient's usual range. During carotid occlusion blood pressure should be maintained at or up to 20% higher than the patient's highest recorded resting blood pressure while awake.
      3. Surgical manipulation of the carotid sinus can cause abrupt bradycardia and hypotension. This may be prevented by infiltration of the sinus with local anesthetic. If infiltration has not been performed, then clamp application may cause hypertension and tachycardia since the sinus is now sensing a low pressure.
      4. Ventilation should be adjusted to maintain normocapnia. Hypocapnia can produces cerebral vasoconstriction. Hypercapnia can induce intracerebral steal phenomenon.
      5. Heparin (5000-10,000 units IV) is usually given prior to occlusion of the carotid artery. Protamine, 50-75 mg, can be given for reversal prior to skin closure.
   D. **Monitoring**
      1. Intraarterial blood pressure monitoring is mandatory.
      2. Additional hemodynamic monitoring should be based primarily on the patients underlying cardiac function. Carotid endarterectomy is not usually associated with significant blood loss or fluid shifts.
      3. Cerebral monitoring
         a. Electroencephalogram and somatosensory evoked potentials (SSEP) have been used to determine the need for a shunt.

122 Vascular Surgery

E. Regional anesthesia

1. Regional anesthesia can be achieved by performing a superficial and deep cervical plexus block, which effectively blocks the C2-C4 nerves. The principal advantage of this technique is that the patient remains awake and can be examined intraoperatively. The need for a temporary shunt can be assessed and any new neurologic deficits diagnosed during surgery.
2. Disadvantages of regional anesthesia include patient discomfort and loss of cooperation, confusion, panic, or seizures. The awkwardness of these possibilities discourages the majority from using the technique.

F. Postoperative considerations

1. Postoperative hypertension may be related to surgical denervation of the ipsilateral carotid baroreceptor. Hypertension can stress and rupture the surgical anastomosis resulting in the development of a wound hematoma, which can rapidly compromise the airway.
2. Transient postoperative hoarseness and ipsilateral deviation of the tongue may occur. They are due to surgical retraction of the recurrent laryngeal and hypoglossal nerves, respectively.

II. Anesthesia for surgery of the aorta

A. Ascending aorta

1. Surgery routinely uses median sternotomy and CPB.
2. Anesthesia is similar to that for cardiac operations involving CPB.
3. The left radial artery should be used to monitor arterial blood pressure, because clamping of the innominate artery maybe necessary during the procedure.

B. Aortic arch.
Usually performed through a median sternotomy with deep hypothermic circulatory arrest. See section on DHCA.

C. Descending thoracic aorta

1. Generally performed through a left thoracotomy without CPB.
2. **Monitoring**
   a. Arterial blood pressure should be monitored from the right radial artery, since clamping of the left subclavian may be necessary.
   b. Pulmonary artery catheter is helpful for following cardiac function and intraoperative fluid management.
3. Cross clamping of the aorta results in a sudden increase in left ventricular afterload which may precipitate acute left ventricular failure or myocardial ischemia in patients with underlying ventricular dysfunction or coronary disease. A nitroprusside infusion is usually required to prevent excessive increases in blood pressure.
4. Release hypotension. following the release of the aortic cross clamp, the abrupt decrease in afterload combined with bleeding and the release of vasodilating acid metabolites from the ischemic lower body can precipitate severe systemic hypotension. Decreasing anesthetic depth, volume loading, and partial or slow release of the cross-clamp may help decrease the severity of hypotension.
5. **Complications**
   a. **Paraplegia.** The incidence of transient postoperative deficits (11%) and postoperative paraplegia (6%).
   b. The classic deficit is that of an anterior spinal artery syndrome with loss of motor function and pinprick sensation but preservation of vibration and proprioception.
   c. **Artery of Adamkiewicz.** This artery has a variable origin from the

aorta, arising between T5 and T8 in 15%, between T9 and T12 in 60%, and between L1 and L2 in 25% of patients.
  d. Measures used to help protect the spinal cord include: use of a temporary heparin coated shunt or partial cardiopulmonary bypass; mild hypothermia; mannitol (related to its ability to lower cerebrospinal pressure by decreasing its production); and drainage of cerebrospinal fluid.
  e. **Renal failure.** Infusion of mannitol (0.5 g/kg) prior to cross-clamping may decrease the incidence of renal failure. Low dose dopamine has not been shown to be as effective but may be used as an adjunct for persistently low urine output.

D. Surgery on the abdominal aorta
  1. Either an anterior transperitoneal or an anterolateral retroperitoneal approach is commonly used.
  2. Monitoring is similar to other aorta surgery..
  3. The aorta cross-clamp is usually applied to the supraceliac, suprarenal, or infrarenal aorta. In general, the farther distally the clamp is applied, the less the effect on left ventricular afterload. Heparinization is necessary prior to cross-clamp.
  4. Release of the aortic clamp frequently produces hypotension. The same techniques to prevent release hypotension as discussed above should be used. Cross-clamp placed at the level of the infrarenal aorta in patients with good ventricular function frequently have minimal hemodynamic changes when the clamp is removed.
  5. Fluid requirements are typically increased (up to 10-12 mL/kg/hr) because of the large incision and extensive retroperitoneal surgical dissection. Fluid requirements should be guided by central venous or pulmonary artery pressure monitoring.
  6. Renal prophylaxis with mannitol should be considered, especially in patients with preexisting renal disease. Clamping of the infrarenal aorta has been shown to significantly decrease renal blood flow, which may contribute to postoperative renal failure.
  7. Epidurals are commonly placed both for intraoperative and postoperative use. The combined technique of epidural and general anesthesia decreases the general anesthetic requirement.

Thoracic Surgery

I. Indications for one-lung anesthesia
A. Absolute
1. Confine pulmonary infection to one side.
2. Confine pulmonary bleeding to one side.
3. Separate ventilation to each lung.
   a. Bronchopulmonary fistula.
   b. Tracheobronchial disruption.
   c. Large lung cyst.
4. Bronchopleural lavage.

B. Relative
1. High priority
   a. Thoracic aortic aneurysm.
   b. Pneumonectomy.
   c. Upper lobectomy.
   d. Thoracoscopy.
2. Low priority
   a. Middle and lower lobectomies.
   b. Sub-segmental resections.
   c. Esophageal surgery.

II. Physiology of one-lung anesthesia
A. One-lung anesthesia results in a large ventilation-perfusion mismatch, secondary to a large intrapulmonary shunt.
B. Factors known to inhibit hypoxic pulmonary vasoconstriction include: (1) very high or very low pulmonary artery pressures; (2) hypocapnia; (3) vasodilators; (4) high or low mixed venous oxygen; (5) pulmonary infection; (6) volatile anesthetics.
C. Factors that decrease blood flow to the ventilated lung: high mean airway pressure; vasoconstrictors; low FIO_2.
D. Carbon dioxide elimination is usually not affected by one-lung anesthesia provide minute ventilation is unchanged.

Preoperative Laboratory Criteria for Pneumonectomy	
Test	High Risk Patient
Arterial Blood Gas	$PaCO_2$ > 45 mmHg (on RA)
FEV_1	< 2 liters
FEV_1/FVC	< 50% of predicated
Maximum Breathing Capacity	< 50% of predicated
RV/TLC	< 50%

Calculation of predicted pulmonary function after pneumonectomy: Predicted postoperative FEV_1 = FEV_1 x perfusion (%) to remaining lung. Calculation of predicted pulmonary function after lobectomy: Loss of function = preoperative FEV_1 x number of functional segments in lobe to be resected divided by the total number of segments in both lungs

III. Management of hypoxia during one-lung anesthesia
  A. Confirm tube placement. Increase oxygen to 100%.
  B. Change tidal volume (8-15 cc/kg) and ventilatory rate.
  C. Periodic inflation of the collapsed lung with 100% oxygen.
  D. Continuous insufflation of oxygen into the collapsed lung.
  E. Adding 5 cm H_2O of continuous positive airway pressure (CPAP) to the collapsed lung.
  F. Adding 5 cm H_2O of positive end expiratory pressure (PEEP) to the ventilated lung.
  G. Adding additional CPAP, followed by additional PEEP.
  H. Early ligation of the ipsilateral pulmonary artery (in a pneumonectomy).

IV. Evaluation of lung resectability
  A. Initial evaluation includes PFTs and arterial blood gas (ABG). If the $PaCO_2$ is above 40 mmHg, the maximum breathing capacity or FEV_1 is below 50%, or the residual volume/total lung capacity is greater than 50%, then split lung function tests should be performed.
  B. Regional pulmonary function test
    1. Regional lung function can be determined by radiospirometry.
    2. The predicted postoperative FEV1 can be calculated by multiplying the preoperative FEV1 by the percent of pulmonary function contributed by the uninvolved lung. The lowest predicted postoperative FEV1 that allows adequate elimination of carbon dioxide is reported to be 800cc.
    3. If the split lung function criteria are not satisfied balloon occlusion of the pulmonary artery ipsilateral to the diseased lung can be performed

Lung Transplantation

I. General information
  A. Indications include end-stage pulmonary parenchymal disease or pulmonary hypertension.
  B. Patients typically have dyspnea at rest or with minimal activity, and resting hypoxemia (PaO2 <50 mmHg) with increasing oxygen requirements.
  C. Organ selection is based on size and ABO compatibility.

II. Anesthetic considerations
  A. Preoperative consideration
    1. These procedures are performed on an emergency basis so patients may have little time to fast for surgery.
    2. Oral cyclosporine is usually given preoperatively (resulting in a full stomach).
    3. Most patients are very sensitive to sedatives.
  B. Intraoperative management
    1. **Monitoring.** In addition to standard ASA monitors, arterial line, central venous pressure monitoring, and pulmonary artery catheter are commonly used.
    2. **Induction/Maintenance**
       a. A modified rapid sequence induction with moderate head-up position is commonly utilized. Hypoxemia and hypercarbia must be avoided to prevent further increases in pulmonary artery pressure.
       b. Methylprednisolone is usually given prior to release of vascular clamps.

C. Postoperative management
1. Patients are left intubated after surgery for 24-72 hours.
2. A thoracic or lumbar epidural may be employed for postoperative analgesia when coagulation studies are normal.

Obstetrical Anesthesia

I. Labor and delivery
A. Stages of labor
1. **First stage.** This stage begins with the onset of regular contractions and ends with full cervical dilation. Pain during the first stage is caused by uterine contractions and cervical dilatation. Pain is carried by the visceral afferent fibers (T10 to L1).
2. **Second stage.** This stage begins with full cervical dilation and ends with delivery of the infant. Pain at the end of the first stage signals the beginning of fetal descent. Pain in the second stage of labor is due to stretching of the birth canal, vulva, and perineum and is conveyed by the afferent fibers of the posterior roots of the S2 to S4 nerves.

B. Physiological changes in pregnancy
1. **Hematological alterations**
   a. Increased plasma volume (40-50%).
   b. Increased total blood volume (25-40%).
   c. Dilutional anemia (hematocrit 35%).
2. **Cardiovascular changes**
   a. Increased cardiac output (30-50%).
   b. Aortocaval compression (supine hypotension syndrome occurs in 10%).
3. **Ventilatory changes**
   a. Increased alveolar ventilation (70%).
   b. Decreased functional residual capacity (20%).
   c. Airway edema.
   d. Decreased PaCO2 (30%).
4. **Gastrointestinal changes**
   a. Prolonged gastric emptying.
   b. Decreased lower esophageal sphincter tone.
5. **Altered drug responses**
   a. Decreased requirements for inhaled anesthetics (MAC).
   b. Decreased local anesthetic requirements.

C. Fetal heart monitoring
1. **Early deceleration.** Related to head compression.
2. **Late deceleration.** Related to uteroplacental insufficiency.
3. **Variable deceleration.** Related to umbilical cord compression.

II. Medications used during labor
A. Vasopressors
Hypotension can result from regional anesthesia, aortocaval compression, or peripartum hemorrhage. **Ephedrine** provides both cardiac stimulation and increased uterine blood flow. Ephedrine is the drug of choice for the treatment of maternal hypotension. **Phenylephrine**, being a pure alpha-adrenergic agent, increases maternal blood pressure at the expense of uteroplacental blood flow.

B. Oxytocin (Pitocin)
1. **Indications.** Oxytocin stimulates uterine contractions and is used to induce or augment labor, to control postpartum bleeding and uterine atony.
2. Oxytocin stimulates both the frequency and force of contractions of uterine smooth muscle. It may cause hypotension, dysrhythmias, and tachycardia.

128 Obstetrical Anesthesia

C. Tocolytics

1. **Indications.** used to delay or stop premature labor, to slow or arrest labor while initiating other therapeutic measures.
2. **Contraindications.** chorioamnionitis, fetal distress, and preeclampsia or eclampsia.
3. **Terbutaline and ritodrine**
   a. Selective beta-2 agonist used to inhibit preterm labor. Beta-2 stimulation also produces bronchodilation and vasodilation and may result in tachycardia. It may cause dysrhythmias, pulmonary edema, hypertension, hypokalemia, or CNS excitement.
   b. **Terbutaline dose.** 10 mcg/min IV infusion. Titrate to a maximum dose of 80 mcg/min.
   c. **Ritodrine dose.** IV infusion of 0.1-0.35 mg/min.
4. **Magnesium sulfate** is used most commonly in preeclampsia, but it is also used as a tocolytic.

III. Anesthesia for labor

A. Systemic medications.
Meperidine, numorphan, butorphanol and nalbuphine are frequently used to relieve pain and anxiety during labor and delivery.

B. Epidural blockade

1. **Epidurals** are placed after the patient is in active labor (5-6 cm dilated in a primipara, 3-4 cm in a multipara).
2. **Preparation before epidural placement**
   a. The patient should be well hydrated first (except PIH patients) with 500-1000 cc of crystalloid solution.
   b. Document baseline vitals (including fetal heart rate).
3. **Epidural opioids for labor**
   a. Fentanyl. 100-200 mcg provides quick onset (5-10 min) but brief duration (1-2 hours).
   b. Sufentanil. 5-15 mcg (mixed in 10 cc preservative free saline) provides relief for about 1-2 hours.
4. **Epidural anesthesia for labor**
   a. Test dose. 3 cc of 1.5% lidocaine with epinephrine (1:200,000) should be given to test for subarachnoid or intravascular placement. Epinephrine should be ommited if the patient has PIH.
   b. Load with 8-15 cc 0.125% bupivacaine with 2 mcg/cc fentanyl followed by a continuous infusion:
      (1) 0.125% bupivacaine at 10-14 cc/hr.
      (2) 0.0625% bupivacaine plus fentanyl 2 mcg/cc at 12-16 cc/hr.
      (3) 0.125% bupivacaine plus sufentanil 0.2 mcg/cc at 10-14 cc/hr.
      (4) 0.0625% bupivacaine plus sufentanil 0.2 mcg/cc at 12-16 cc/hr.
   c. Infusion rates are commonly adjusted as labor progresses. Bolus local anesthetic or narcotic (fentanyl 50-100 mcg) can also be given as needed.
   d. Blood pressure should be monitored every few minutes for 20-30 minutes and every 15 minutes thereafter.

C. Intrathecal opioids for labor

1. Intrathecal opioids can be used for multiparas in very active labor (6-9 cm) or primiparas who are fully dilated with significant pain. They can also be used for patients in early labor, 2-4 cm dilated, prior to active phase.
2. Fentanyl. 25 mcg fentanyl in 1 cc preservative free saline provides

about 1 hour of analgesia.
3. **Meperidine.** 10-20 mg provides about 2 hours of analgesia.
4. **Sufentanil.** 10 mcg in 1-2 cc preservative free saline provides about 3 hours of analgesia.

D. Spinal anesthesia for labor
1. Saddle block can be used if a forceps delivery is required or in the postpartum period, for repair of traumatic lacerations of the vagina or rectum or for removal of retained placenta.
2. After prehydrating the patient, sufentanil 10 mcg or fentanyl 25 mcg with bupivacaine 1.25-2.5 mg may be used. Hyperbaric 5% lidocaine 40-50 mg can also be used.

E. Combined spinal-epidural for labor
1. Combined spinal/epidural may be useful for patients presenting in early labor because the spinal can be given to help with early labor pain, while the epidural can be activated after the patient is in active labor.
2. Spinal. 25 mcg fentanyl in 1 cc saline or 10 mcg Sufenta in 1 cc saline.
3. An epidural is initiated as noted above after the pain returns.

IV. Cesarean section

A. Anesthetic management
1. All patients should have a wedge under the right hip for left uterine displacement (15 degrees). All patients should receive Bicitra 30 cc PO (metoclopramide 10 mg IV is optional).
2. All patients (except PIH patients) should be hydrated before the block is placed.
3. Pre-op labs. Hematocrit, hemoglobin, clot to blood bank (for crash cesarean section hematocrit). Patients with PIH should receive a PT/PTT, platelet, and bleeding time done prior to epidural/spinal.
4. Treat hypotension with fluids and ephedrine to maintain systolic blood pressure >100.
5. After placenta delivered, oxytocin 20-40 units should be added to IV fluids (if uterine bleeding does not decrease, methergine 0.2 mg IM may be given).

B. Epidural anesthesia
1. **Initial dose.** 1.5-2% lidocaine with/without epinephrine, 0.5% bupivacaine or 3% chloroprocaine may be used (most commonly use 20-25 cc 2% lidocaine with epinephrine). For rapid onset, sodium bicarbonate, 1 cc for each 10 cc of local anesthetic, can be added. Administer 20 cc (in 3-5cc increments) to obtain T2-T4 level. Rebolus as necessary.
2. **Fentanyl.** 50-100 mcg will speed the onset of action, potentiate intraoperative analgesia, decrease nausea and vomiting during uterine manipulation, decrease requirements for supplemental opioid medication, and reduce shivering.
3. **Post-op pain control.** Duramorph 3-5 mg epidurally, given after the umbilical cord is clamped, provides 18-24 hours of postoperative pain relief.

C. Spinal anesthesia
1. **Bupivacaine** 0.75% in 8.25% dextrose 8-15 mg is the most commonly used local anesthetic.
2. **Fentanyl.** 10-25 mcg speeds the onset of action, potentiates intraoperative analgesia, decreases nausea and vomiting during uterine manipulation, decreases requirements for supplemental opioid

130 Obstetrical Anesthesia

   medication, reduces shivering.
   3. **Duramorph.** 0.10-0.25 mg provides 18-24 hours of postoperative pain relief.
- **D.** If the block becomes "patchy" prior to delivery of the baby, should be treated with ketamine, 10-20 mg IV, or 30% nitrous; after delivery, an IV narcotic may be used.
- **E. General anesthesia** is generally reserved for emergency cesarean sections when regional anesthesia is refused or contraindicated, when substantial hemorrhage is anticipated, or when uterine relaxation is required.
    1. General anesthesia allows for rapid induction, control of airway, and decreased incidence of hypotension. Aspiration and failed intubation remain a major cause of morbidity and mortality.
    2. **Technique**
        a. Patients should be premedicated with Bicitra, 30 cc, metoclopramide 10 mg, and cimetidine, 300 mg, or ranitidine, 50 mg.
        b. Preoxygenate with 100% oxygen for 3 minutes if time allows or 5-6 deep breaths.
        c. Rapid-sequence induction with cricoid pressure is performed with thiopental 4-5 mg/kg (ketamine 1 mg/kg for asthmatics and hemodynamically unstable patients) and succinylcholine 1.5 mg/kg.
        d. Anesthesia is maintained with a 50% mixture of nitrous and oxygen, combined with a volatile agent (enflurane 0.5-0.75% or isoflurane 0.75%). Hyperventilation should be avoided because of adverse effects on uterine blood flow.
        e. Oxytocin (10-40 units/l) is added to the IV infusion after delivery of the placenta to stimulate uterine contraction.
        f. After the baby is delivered, a muscle relaxant may be administered (usually one dose of atracurium, 0.5 mg/kg, or vecuronium, 0.05 mg/kg), fentanyl 100-150 mcg, versed 1-2 mg, nitrous 70%/oxygen 30%, and discontinue inhalation agent.
        g. Prior to extubation an orogastric tube should be passed to empty the stomach.

V. Pregnancy induced hypertension (PIH)

- **A.** Preeclampsia is characterized by hypertension (SBP >140 or DBP >90) or a consistent increase in SBP by 30 or DBP by 15, proteinuria (> 500 mg/day), and generalized edema occurring after the 20th week of gestation and resolving within 48 hours after delivery). 5-7% incidence in pregnancy, occurring mostly in young primigravidas.
- **B. Predisposing factors.** Multiple gestation, major uterine anomalies, chronic hypertension, chronic renal disease, diabetes, polyhydramnios, molar pregnancy, fetal hydrops.
- **C. Severe PIH** is defined as BP > 160/110, pulmonary edema, proteinuria >5 gm/day, oliguria, central nervous system manifestations, hepatic tenderness, or HEELP syndrome.
- **D. Pathophysiologic alterations**
    1. **Hematologic.** Decrease in intravascular volume (primarily plasma), disseminated intravascular coagulation characterized initially by reduction in platelets; later by rise in fibrin degradation products, fall in fibrinogen level, increased PT/PTT.
    2. **Cerebral.** Hyperreflexia, CNS irritability increase, coma, increased intracranial pressure, altered consciousness.

3. **Respiratory.** Upper airway and laryngeal edema.
4. **Cardiac.** Arteriolar constriction and increase of peripheral resistance leading to increased BP.
5. **Ophthalmic.** Retinal arteriolar spasm, blurred vision, retinal edema and possible retina detachment.
6. **Renal.** Reduction in renal blood flow and GFR, elevated plasma uric acid (increased levels correlate with severity of disease), deposition of fibrin in glomeruli.
7. **Hepatic.** Elevated LFTs, hepatocellular damage or edema secondary to vasospasm, epigastric or right upper quadrant abdominal pain.

F. Management
1. **Definitive therapy** includes delivery of fetus and the placenta with symptoms usually resolving within 48 hours.
2. **Antihypertensive drugs.** Hydralazine is the agent of choice because it increases both uteroplacental and renal blood flow. Labetalol can also be used. Continuous infusions of nitroprusside can be used in treating hypertensive crisis or acute increases in blood pressure.
3. **Fluid management.** Fluids are generally not restricted. Intravascular depletion should be corrected with crystalloids.
4. **Magnesium therapy.** Magnesium sulfate is a mild vasodilator and central nervous system depressant. Give 2-4 gram loading dose (slow IV over 5-15 minutes), followed by continuous infusion of 1-3 grams/hour. Therapeutic maternal blood levels of 4-8 mEq/l should be maintained

G. Anesthetic management
1. All patients should have a bleeding time, platelet count, coagulation profile, CBC, Mg level, fibrinogen, fibrin split products, lytes, uric acid level, and LFTs prior to anesthesia.
2. **Indications for invasive monitoring**
   a. Unresponsive or refractory hypertension: increased systemic vascular resistance or increased cardiac output.
   b. Pulmonary edema. Cardiogenic or left ventricular failure, increased systemic vascular resistance, or noncardiogenic volume overload.
   c. Persistent arterial desaturation.
   d. Oliguria unresponsive to modest fluid loading: low preload, severe increased systemic vascular resistance with low cardiac output, selective renal artery vasoconstriction.
   e. Other orders and medications: patients should have blood pressure under control before (DBP<110) starting epidural. Epidural anesthesia is the preferred method of analgesia for vaginal delivery and cesarean section in most patients including those with eclampsia. Spinal can be used. General anesthetics are reserved for fetal distress, coagulopathies or hypovolemia.

H. HELLP syndrome
1. HELLP syndrome. Hemolysis, elevated liver enzymes, low platelets.
2. Occurs in 4-12% of severe PIH patients.
3. Reported perinatal mortality: 7.7-60%. Maternal mortality 3.5-24.2%.
4. Diagnostic criteria. Platelet count less than 100,000/mm^3, hemolysis by peripheral smear and increased bilirubin greater than 1.2 mg/dl, SGOT greater than 70 U/L and LDH greater than 600 U/L.
5. High incidence of maternal complications including abruptio placenta, coagulopathy (DIC, prolonged PT and PTT), acute renal failure, ruptured hepatic hematoma.

132 Obstetrical Anesthesia

VI. Peripartum hemorrhage
   A. **Placenta previa.** Abnormal implantation of the placenta in the lower uterine segment; incidence is 0.1-1.0% (higher in subsequent pregnancies); presents with painless vaginal bleeding; potential for massive blood loss; risk factors include prior uterine scar, prior placenta previa, advanced maternal age, and multiparity.
   B. **Abruptio placentae.** Premature separation of a normally implanted placenta; incidence is 0.2-2.4% (predisposing conditions: hypertension, uterine abnormalities, history of cocaine abuse); presents with painful vaginal bleeding, abnormalities in fetal heart rate, irritable uterus; potential for massive blood loss (blood loss may be concealed), disseminated intravascular coagulation (DIC), renal failure.
   C. **Uterine rupture.** Incidence: 0.008-0.1% (predisposing conditions: previous uterine surgery, prolonged intrauterine manipulation); may presents with sudden onset of breakthrough pain (although most patients with uterine rupture have no pain) with or without vaginal bleeding, abnormalities in fetal heart rate, irritable uterus; potential for massive blood loss.
   D. **Vasa previa.** A condition in which the umbilical card of the fetus passes in front of the presenting part making them vulnerable to trauma during vaginal examination or during artificial rupture of membranes. Bleeding here is from the fetal circulation only.
   E. **Retained placenta.** Incidence is about 1% of all vaginal deliveries and usually requires manual exploration of the uterus. If uterine relaxation is required, and bleeding is minimal, nitroglycerin, 50-100 mcg boluses, can be given. Small doses of ketamine may be used if a regional anesthetic is not in place.
   F. **Uterine atony.** Occurs in 2-5% of patients. Treatment includes oxytocin, or if this fails, one of the other oxytocics.
   G. **Laceration** of the vagina, cervix or perineum is very common.
   H. **Uterine inversion** is very rare and is a true obstetrical emergency. General anesthesia is generally required to allow immediate uterine relaxation. These patients can exsanguinate rapidly.

VII. Anesthesia for nonobstetric surgery during pregnancy
   A. Approximately 1-2% of pregnant patients require surgery during their pregnancy. Maternal morbidity and mortality is unchanged from that of nonpregnant women, but fetal mortality ranges from 5-35%.
   B. Nitrous oxide and benzodiazepines have been linked to congenital anomalies and should be avoided. Regional anesthesia should be used when possible to minimize fetal exposure. Fetal heart rate and uterine activity should be monitored with a Doppler and tocodynamometer after the 16th week of gestation.

Neuroanesthesia

I. Cerebrospinal fluid (CSF)
   A. Produced at a rate of 0.3 cc/min (about 21 cc/hr or 500 cc/day) primarily by the choroid plexuses of the cerebral (mainly lateral) ventricles. Smaller amounts are formed directly by ependymal cell linings and yet smaller amounts from fluid leaking into the perivascular spaces surrounding cerebral vessels (blood-brain barrier leakage). CSF is reabsorbed at a rate of 0.3-0.4 cc/min into the venous system by the villi in the arachnoid membrane.
   B. CSF production is decreased by carbonic anhydrase inhibitors (acetazolamide), corticosteroids, spironolactone, loop diuretics (furosemide), isoflurane, and vasoconstrictors.
   C. Cerebral spinal fluid volume: 100-150 ml normal.

II. Cerebral blood flow
   A. **Cerebral blood flow rates**
   1. Cerebral blood flow averages 50 ml/100 gm/min (gray matter is about 80 ml/100 gm/min and white matter is about 20 ml/100 gm/min). Total cerebral blood flow in adults averages 750 cc/min (15-20% of cardiac output).
   2. Flow rates below 20-25 cc/100 g/min are usually associated with cerebral impairment (slowing of EEG).
   3. Cerebral blood flow rates between 15 and 20 cc/100 g/min produce a flat (isoelectric) EEG.
   4. Cerebral blood flow rates below 10 cc/100 g/min are usually associated with irreversible brain damage.

   B. **Cerebral blood flow determinants**
   1. $PaCO_2$: For every 1 mmHg change in $PaCO_2$ from there is a corresponding change in CBF by 1-2 ml/100 g/min. Cerebral blood flow is directly proportionate to $PaCO_2$ between tensions of 20 and 80 mmHg.
   2. PaO_2: No significant increase in CBF until below 50 mmHg.
   3. Temperature. Cerebral blood flow changes 5-7% per degree Celsius. Hypothermia decreases both cerebral metabolic and cerebral blood flow.
   4. Cerebral perfusion pressure autoregulation. CPP = MAP - CVP (or ICP if greater), chronic hypertension shifts the autoregulation curve to the right; autoregulation is impaired in presence of intracranial tumors or volatile anesthetics.
   5. Anesthetic drugs. Volatile agents are potent cerebral vasodilators (halothane > enflurane > isoflurane), ketamine and nitrous oxide are cerebral vasodilators (opioids, benzodiazepines, and barbiturates are cerebral vasoconstrictors).
   6. Hematocrit. CBF increases with decreasing viscosity (hematocrit). Optimal cerebral oxygen delivery occurs at hematocrits between 30-34%.
   7. Regionally, CBF and metabolism are tightly coupled. An increase in cortical activity will lead to a corresponding increase in CBF.
   8. Sympathetic tone does not appreciably affect CBF.
   9. Intracranial components are brain bulk (80%), blood volume (5%), and CSF (15%). A small increase in intracranial volume can be partially compensated by translocation of CSF into the spinal subarachnoid space and compression on the venous blood volume. This compensa-

tion mechanism is limited, and once exhausted, any further increase in volume will lead to a rise in ICP.

III. Cerebral metabolism
A. The brain receives 15% of the cardiac output and consumes 20% of the oxygen.

B. Temperature. Cerebral metabolic rate decreases 7% for every 1 degree Celsius reduction in temperature.

C. Cerebral metabolic rate for oxygen averages 3.0-3.5 ml/100 gm/min. Cerebral metabolic rate ($CMRO_2$) is greatest in the gray matter of the cerebral cortex and generally parallels cortical electrical activity.

D. Luxury perfusion. Describes the combination of a decrease in neuronal metabolic demand with an increase in cerebral blood flow (metabolic supply). This altered coupling of cerebral blood flow and cerebral metabolic rate occurs with volatile agents.

IV. Intracranial pressure (ICP)
A. Normal ICP is 5-10 mmHg.

B. Intracranial hypertension is defined as a sustained increase in ICP above 15 mmHg.

C. When intracranial pressure exceeds 30 mmHg, cerebral blood flow progressively decreases and a vicious cycle is established: ischemia causes brain edema, which in turn increases intracranial pressure, resulting in more ischemia.

D. Periodic increases in arterial blood pressure with reflex slowing of the heart rate (Cushing response) are often observed and can be correlated with abrupt increases in intracranial pressure lasting 1-15 minutes.

E. Cerebral perfusion pressure (CPP) = MAP - ICP (or central venous pressure (CVP), whichever is greater).

F. Compensatory mechanisms for increased ICP
  1. Displacement of CSF from the cranial to the spinal compartment.
  2. Increase in CSF absorption.
  3. Decrease in CSF production.
  4. Decrease in total cerebral blood volume (primarily venous).

G. Evidence of increased intracranial pressure
  1. Symptoms. Nausea/vomiting, mental status changes (drowsiness progressing to coma), personality changes, visual changes, neck stiffness, focal deficits, hypertension, bradycardia, absent brain stem reflexes, decerebrate posturing, fixed and dilated pupils, respiratory rhythm changes (irregular rhythm or apnea).
  2. Signs. Headache, papilledema, posturing, bulging fontanelles in infants, seizures, altered patterns of breathing, cushing's reflex (hypertension and bradycardia).
  3. **Radiologic Signs**
     a. X-ray. Suture separation, erosion of clinoid process, copper-beaten skull.
     b. CT/MRI Scans. Midline shift, cerebral edema, mass lesions, abnormal ventricular size, obliteration of basal cistern.
  4. **Cushing reflex**
     a. **Cushing reflex.** Periodic increases in arterial blood pressure with reflex slowing of the heart is the Cushing response and often observed and correlated with abrupt increases in intracranial pressure (plateau or A waves) lasting 1-15 minutes.
     b. **Cushing triad.** Hypertension, bradycardia, respiratory disturbances (late and unreliable sign that usually just proceeds brain

herniation).
   c. Continued profound sympathetic nervous system (SNS) discharge during Cushing's reflex may hide a state of hypovolemia. If the Cushing source is taken away by surgical intervention and/or the SNS response is ablated by anesthesia, one may encounter profound and resistant hypotension.
5. **Treatment of elevated ICP**
   a. **Reduce cerebral blood volume**
      (1) Hyperventilation ($PaCO_2$ 20-25 mmHg). Excessive hyperventilation ($PaCO_2$ <20) may cause cerebral ischemia.
      (2) Prevent straining or coughing on the endotracheal tube.
      (3) Elevation of the head to encourage venous drainage.
   b. **Reduce cerebrospinal fluid volume**
      (1) Ventriculostomy or lumbar subarachnoid catheter.
      (2) Decrease CSF production with acetazolamide.
      (3) Recent studies suggest that administration of hypertonic saline and mannitol reduce the production of CSF and may contribute to the immediate effect of ICP reduction.
      (4) Reduce brain volume by decreasing brain water with osmotic diuretics (20% mannitol 0.25 - 1.0 g/kg); mannitol is thought to reduce cerebral swelling by osmotic dehydration, loop diuretics (furosemide 0.5 mg/kg), and steroids (decadron).
      (5) Barbiturates are potent cerebral vasoconstrictors that decrease cerebral blood volume while decreasing cerebral metabolic rate.

V. Methods of cerebral protection
A. **Barbiturates**, etomidate, propofol, and isoflurane may offer protection against focal ischemia and incomplete global ischemia by producing complete electrical silence of the brain and eliminated the metabolic cost of electrical activity; unfortunately, they have no effect on basal energy requirements.
B. **Hypothermia**
   1. Cerebral metabolic rate is decreased by 7% for every 1 degree Celsius reduction in temperature.
   2. Hypothermia decreases both basal and electrical metabolic requirements throughout the brain; metabolic requirement continue to decrease even after complete electrical silence.
   3. Hypothermia is the most effective method for protecting the brain during focal and global ischemia.
C. The calcium channel blockers, nimodipine and nicardipine, may be beneficial in reducing neurologic injury following hemorrhagic and ischemic strokes.
D. Maintenance of optimal cerebral perfusion pressure is critical (maintaining normal arterial blood pressure, intracranial pressure, oxygen carrying capacity, and arterial oxygen tension; hematocrit should be maintained 30-34%). Hyperglycemia has aggravates neurologic injuries and should be avoided.

VI. Pharmacology
A. **Inhalational anesthetics**
   1. Halothane, enflurane, desflurane, sevoflurane and isoflurane produce dose-dependent decreases in $CMRO_2$ and uncouple $CMRO_2$ from CBF.
   2. Enflurane increases CSF formation and retard absorption. Halothane

136 Neuroanesthesia

impedes CSF absorption but only minimally retards formation.
- **B.** Most intravenous agents cause coupled reduction in CBF and $CMRO_2$ in a dose-dependent manner. Ketamine is the only intravenous anesthetic that dilates the cerebral vasculature and increases CBF.
- **C.** All muscle relaxants, except succinylcholine, have no direct effect on CBF and $CMRO_2$. Succinylcholine causes a transient increase in CBF and $CMRO_2$.

VII. Anesthesia for Craniotomy
- **A. Preoperative Preparation**
    1. Preanesthetic evaluation should establish the presence or absence of intracranial hypertension.
    2. Physical examination should include a neurologic assessment documenting mental status and any existing sensory or motor deficits.
    3. Computerized tomography (CT) and MRI scans should be reviewed for evidence of brain edema, a midline shift greater than 0.5 cm, and ventricular size.
    4. Premedication
        - **a.** Premedication is best avoided when intracranial hypertension is suspected.
        - **b.** Corticosteroids and anticonvulsant therapy should be continued up until the time of surgery.
- **B. Monitoring**
    1. In addition to standard ASA monitors, direct intraarterial pressure monitoring and bladder catheterization are indicated for most patients undergoing craniotomy.
    2. Central venous access and pressure monitoring should be considered for patients requiring vasoactive drugs.
- **C. Induction and maintenance of anesthesia**
    1. Induction must be accomplished without increasing ICP or compromising CBF. Hypertension, hypotension, hypoxia, hypercarbia, and coughing should also be avoided.
    2. Thiopental, propofol, Etomidate may be used for IV induction and may be supplemented by midazolam and opioids.
    3. Nondepolarizing agents are the muscle relaxants of choice. The hemodynamic response to laryngoscopy can be blunted by pretreatment with lidocaine, labetalol, opioids, and/or esmolol.
    4. Anesthesia is usually maintained with a combination of a opioid, volatile agent, and muscle relaxant. Anesthetic requirements are decreased after craniotomy and dural opening, since the brain parenchyma is devoid of sensation.
- **D. Emergence** should occur slow and controlled. Straining, coughing and hypertension should be avoided. Patients left intubated should remain sedated.

VIII. Head trauma
- **A. Glasgow Coma Scale** (GCS) correlates with the severity of injury and outcome. Total score possible = 3-15.
    1. Best motor response. 6-obeys commands; 5-localizes pain; 4-withdrawals; 3-flexion: decorticate rigidity; 2-extension: decerebrate rigidity; 1-no motor response.
    2. Best verbal response: 5-oriented, conversant; 4-disoriented, conversant; 3-inappropriate words; 2-incomprehensible sounds; 1-no verbalization/response.
    3. Eye opening: 4-spontaneous; 3-to verbal stimulation; 2-to pain; 1-no

response.
- **B. Cushing triad.** Hypertension, bradycardia, respiratory disturbances (late and unreliable sign that usually just proceeds brain herniation).
- **C. Preoperative**
  1. All patients should be regarded as having a full stomach and treated as such.
  2. Hypotension in the setting of head trauma is nearly always related to other associated injuries. Correction of hypotension and control of any bleeding take precedence over radiographic studies and definitive neurological treatment because systolic arterial blood pressures of less than 80 mmHg correlate with a poor outcome.
  3. Dysrhythmias and electrocardiographic abnormalities in the T wave, U wave, ST segment, and QT interval are common following head injuries but are not necessarily associated with cardiac injury.
  4. Intraoperative
     a. Anesthetic management is similar to other mass lesions with intracranial hypertension.
     b. Cerebral perfusion pressure should be maintained between 70 and 110 mmHg.
     c. Dextrose containing solutions may exacerbate ischemic brain damage and should be avoided in the absence of documented hypoglycemia.

IX. Spinal cord injury

- **A.** Lesions involving phrenic nerve (C3-C5) usually result in apnea requiring intubation and mechanical ventilatory support. Lesions below C5-C6 may cause up to 70% reduction in vital capacity and FEV, with impaired ventilation and oxygenation. Lesions involving T1-T4 (cardiac accelerator nerves) may lead to bradycardia, bradydysrhythmias, atrioventricular block and cardiac arrest. T7 or higher is the critical level for significant alveolar ventilation impairment.
- **B.** Spinal shock is seen in high spinal cord injuries lasting from a few hours to several weeks; characterized by loss of sympathetic tone in capacitance and resistance vessels below the level of the lesion; flaccid paralysis; total absence of visceral and somatic sensation below level of injury; paralytic ileus; loss of spinal cord reflexes below level of injury.
- **C.** Autonomic hyperreflexia is associated with lesions above T5, not a problem during acute management (appears following resolution of spinal shock and return of spinal cord reflexes).
- **D.** Methylprednisolone: 30 mg/kg IV loading dose, followed by 5.4 mg/kg/hr for 23 hours may improve the functional recovery if treatment is begun within 8 hrs following injury.
- **E.** Succinylcholine: safe for use during the first 24-48 hours.

Pain Management

Pain Management: Patient Controlled Analgesia

Drug	Bolus Dose (mg)	Lockout Interval (min)	Continuous Infusion (mg/hr)
Fentanyl	0.015-0.05	3-10	0.02-0.1
Hydromorphone	0.1-0.5	5-15	0.2-0.5
Meperidine	35,929	5-15	5-40
Methadone	0.5-3.0	10-20	
Morphine	0.5-3.0	5-20	0.5-10
Oxymorphone	0.2-0.8	5-15	0.1-1.0
Sufentanil	0.003-0.015	3-10	0.004-0.03
Pentazocine	35,944	5-15	6-40

Intrathecal Opioids

Opioid	Dose	Onset (min)	Duration (hr)
Morphine	0.15-0.6 mg	15-45	8-24
Fentanyl	10-25 mcg	2-5	1-3
Sufentanil	5-15 mcg	2-5	2-4

Epidural Opioids for Postoperative Analgesia

Drug	Bolus Dose	Onset (min)	Peak (min)	Duration (hr)	Concentration	Rate (ml/hr)
Meperidine	30-100 mg	35,924	12-30	4-6	1 mg/cc	10-20
Morphine	5 mg	23.5	30-60	12-24	0.1 mg/cc	1-6
Methadone	5 mg	12.5	17	7.2		
Hydromorphone	1 mg	13	23	11.4	0.05 mg/cc	6-8
Fentanyl	100 mcg	35,894	20	2.6	4 mcg/cc	4-12
Diamorphine	5 mg	5	9-15	12.4		

Pain Management

Drug	Bolus Dose	Onset (min)	Peak (min)	Duration (hr)	Concentration	Rate (ml/hr)
Sufentanil	30-50 mcg	7.3	26.5	3.9		
Alfentanil	15 mcg/kg	15		1-2		

Continuous Epidural Infusion Analgesia

Bupivacaine (%)	Opioid (concentration)	Infusion Rate (ml/hr)
0.125	Fentanyl 2 mcg/cc	35,892
0.125	Sufentanil 1 mcg/cc	4-8
0.125	Morphine 0.05 mg/cc	4-8
0.0625	Fentanyl 5 mcg/cc	4-10
0.0625	Sufentanil 2 mcg/cc	4-8
0.0625	Morphine 0.1 mg/cc	2-8
	Morphine 0.1 mg/cc	2-8
	Hydromorphone 0.02 mg/cc	1-6

Pain Management: Selected Opioid Analgesic Preparations

Drug	Dose (Adult)
Butorphanol Tartrate (Stadol)	1-2 mg IV q3-4 hr or 2 mg IM q3-4 hr
Codeine	15-60 mg po q4-6 hr
Hydromorphone HCL (Dilaudid)	2 mg q4-6 hr po or 1-2 mg q4-6 hr SC/IM
Morphine (MS Contin)	30-60 mg q12 hr po
Nalbuphine HCL (Nubain)	10 mg q3-4 hr SC, IM, or IV
Oxycodone HCL	5 mg q6 hr po
Oxymorphone (Numorphan)	1-1.5 mg q4-6 hr SC or IM
Propoxyphene HCL (Darvon)	65 mg q4 hr po (cap)

Pain Management: Nonsteroidal Anti-Inflammatory Drugs

Generic Name	Dose	Comments
Acetaminophen	325-650 mg q4-6h PO	Hepatic toxicity follows large doses
Aspirin	325-650 mg q4-6h PO	May cause dyspepsia and GI bleeding, decrease platelet function; less hepatic and renal toxicity
Diflunisal	200-500 mg q8-12h PO	Less irritating to GI tract
Ibuprofen	200-400 mg q8-12h PO	Fewer GI symptoms
Indomethacin	25-50 mg q8h PO	Not recommended in chronic benign pain
Ketorolac	10 mg q6h PO (see pharm section for IV dosing	For acute exacerbations of chronic pain
Naproxen	500 mg initially, then 250 mg q6-8h PO	Slightly more toxic than ibuprofen regarding GI and CNS effects

Postoperative Pain Management

I. **Benefits of epidural analgesia**
   A. Superior pain relief, decreased incidence of pulmonary complications, decreased incidence of cardiovascular complications, earlier return of bowel function.

II. **Clinical pharmacology of epidural opioids**
   A. **Hydrophilic opioids** (morphine, hydromorphone)
      1. Properties. Slow onset, long duration, high CSF solubility, extensive CSF spread.
      2. Advantages. Prolonged single-dose analgesia, thoracic analgesia with lumbar administration, minimal dose compared to IV administration.
      3. Disadvantages. delayed onset of analgesia, unpredictable duration, higher incidence of side effects, delayed respiratory depression.
   B. **Lipophilic opioids** (fentanyl, sufentanil)
      1. Properties. Rapid onset, short duration, low CSF solubility, minimal CSF spread.
      2. Advantages. Rapid analgesia, decreased side effects, ideal for continuous infusion or PCEA.
      3. Disadvantages. Systemic absorption, brief single-dose analgesia, limited thoracic analgesia with lumbar administration.

III. **Epidural placement for postop local anesthetic administration**
   A. Thoracotomy: T4-T6.
   B. Upper abdominal/flank: T8.
   C. Lower abdominal: T10-T12.
   D. Lower extremity/pelvic: L2-L4.

IV. **Side effects of peridural administered opioids**
   A. **Nausea/vomiting.** Opioids in the vomiting center and the chemoreceptor trigger zone in the medulla can cause nausea or vomiting.

B. Pruritus. Although histamine release may play a small role, the cause of pruritus is unknown.

C. Respiratory depression
1. Patients at risk for respiratory depression are the elderly; patients who receive concomitant systemic opiates or sedatives; and patients who have received large doses of spinal opiates.
2. Early respiratory depression can occur within two hours of spinal opioid administration and is similar to that observed with parenteral administration of an opioid. With hydrophilic agents (ie, morphine), late respiratory depression commonly peaks at 12 or 13 hours after the initial dose but can occur as late as 24 hours.
3. Urinary retention.
4. Delayed gastric emptying.

V. Management of opioid related side effects
A. Nausea/vomiting
1. Metoclopramide (Reglan): 10-20 mg IV q4 hrs; low incidence of side effects.
2. Droperidol (Inapsine): 0.625 mg IV q4 hrs; can cause dysphoria, hypotension.

B. Pruritus
1. Naloxone (Narcan): 10-40 mcg/hr IV continuous infusion; will not significantly reverse analgesia at recommended doses.
2. Diphenhydramine (Benadryl): 25-50 mg IV q4 hrs; significant sedative effect.

C. Respiratory depression
1. Naloxone (Narcan). 40-100 mcg/bolus titrated q2-3 minutes; larger than necessary dosage may result in significant reversal of analgesia, nausea, vomiting, sweating, and/or circulatory stress.

D. Urinary retention. Foley as needed.

Trauma

I. **Initial survey and resuscitation**
   A. **Five rules of trauma**
      1. The stomach is always full.
      2. The cervical spine is always unstable.
      3. Altered mental status is caused by head injury.
      4. Partial airway obstruction may progress rapidly to complete airway obstruction.
      5. The patient is always hypovolemic.
   B. **Airway and breathing**
      1. All patients should have initial stabilization of the cervical spine before any airway manipulation. Assume a cervical spine injury in any patient with multi-system trauma, especially with an altered level of consciousness or a blunt injury above the clavicle. Maintain the cervical spine in a neutral position with inline stabilization when establishing an airway.
      2. The airway should be assessed for patency. All secretions, blood, vomitus, and foreign bodies should be removed. Measures to establish a patent airway should protect the cervical spine. The chin lift or jaw thrust maneuvers are recommended to achieve this task.
      3. Establish a patent airway
      4. All patients should receive supplemental oxygen (face mask, bag-valve mask, endotracheal tube).
      5. Patients who arrive intubated, should have placement confirmed (ie, bilateral breath sounds with good chest rise, direct laryngoscopy, or capnography).
   C. **Circulation**
      1. Hypotension following injury must be considered to be hypovolemic in origin until proven otherwise. Volume resuscitation begins immediately with the establishment of intravenous access.
      2. A minimum of two large-caliber intravenous catheters should be established. Blood and fluid warmers should be used.

II. **Trauma intubations**
   A. **Indications for airway intervention**
      1. Airway obstruction.
      2. Hypoxia and hypercarbia (ie, shock or cardiac arrest).
      3. Controlled hyperventilation (patients with obvious intracranial injury or GCS of less than 9).
      4. Protection against pulmonary aspiration (ie, drug overdose).
      5. Airway injury (eg, inhalation injuries).
      6. Sedation for diagnostic procedures (patients who are intoxicated or suffering from possible head injury that are unable to lie still for necessary diagnostic studies).
      7. Prophylactic intubation (patients with impending respiratory failure or airway compromise).
      8. Airway or midface injuries.
      9. Large flail segment.
   B. **Preparation**
      1. All multiple trauma patients should be assumed to have a cervical spine injury and a full stomach. Portable cervical spine x-rays will miss 5% to 15% of injuries. Complete evaluation of the cervical spine may require a CT scan or multiple radiographs and clinical exam. Cervical

spine injury is unlikely in alert patients without neck pain or tenderness.
   2. Patients who arrive ventilated with an esophageal obturator airway (EOA) should have a more definitive airway placed before the EOA is removed. After the trachea has been intubated, the stomach should be suctioned prior to the removal of the EOA.
   3. In alert patients with potential spinal cord injuries, document any movement of extremities before and after intubation.
- C. Airway assessment
   1. The airway should be examined to detect potentially difficult intubation.
   2. Airway equipment (laryngoscope, endotracheal tubes, suction) should be set-up prior to the patients arrival.
- D. Endotracheal intubation
   1. **Preoxygenation**
      a. Preoxygenation helps prevent hypoxia during intubation. All patients should be preoxygenated.
      b. Administration of 100% oxygen to an individual with normal spontaneous ventilation for 3 minutes or 4-6 vital capacity breaths will generally result in 95%-98% nitrogen washout.
   2. **Orotracheal intubation**, facilitated by the use of muscle relaxants and general anesthesia, is the technique of choice for intubating the trachea of trauma patients.
   3. **Nasotracheal intubation**
      a. Contraindications to nasotracheal intubation include: apnea; upper airway foreign body, abscess, or tumor; nasal obstruction; central facial fractures; acute epiglottitis (blind technique); basal skull fractures; coagulopathy; and cardiac or other prosthesis.
   4. **Cricothyroidotomy:** The need for cricothyroidotomy due to severe maxillofacial trauma or an inability to perform oral-tracheal intubation occurs in less than 1% of all trauma patients requiring intubation on admission. It may be used as a primary airway, with injuries to the pharynx for example, or after failure of orotracheal intubation. It may be a full surgical approach or via a percutaneous needle cricothyroidotomy with high flow oxygen.
   5. If there is difficulty or delay in intubating the trachea in any trauma patient with respiratory comprise, a tracheotomy or cricothyroidotomy should be performed immediately.

III. Intraoperative management
- A. Two functioning large bore IVs should be placed before induction. Blood should be available before incision is made, if possible.
- B. Induction
   1. All trauma patients should be assumed to have full stomachs.
   2. When general anesthesia is planned, rapid sequence induction with cricoid pressure is the method of choice.
   3. Reduced doses of induction agent or no induction agent may be appropriate in severely injured, obtunded patients.
- C. Maintenance
   1. Narcotic based anesthetic is recommended for stable patients. For unstable patients, scopolamine/oxygen/pancuronium can be used. Prophylactic use of scopolamine (0.1-0.2 mg IVP) or midazolam (1-3 mg IVP) may be considered.
   2. Small incremental doses of anesthetic agents should be used in patients in shock. Avoid using nitrous oxide.

3. The patient should be kept warm. All patients should have a blanket warmer, fluid warmer, and a bear hugger on the upper body or lower body. Hypothermia worsens acid-base disorders, coagulopathies, and myocardial function.

IV. Burns

A. Preoperative evaluation
1. First-degree burns are limited to the epithelium, while second-degree burns extend into the dermis, and third-degree burns destroy the entire skin thickness.
2. The size of the burn should be estimated as a percentage of the total body surface area (%TBSA).
3. Indications for early intubation include hypoxemia not correctable with oxygen by face mask, upper airway edema, or the presence of copious secretions.

B. Perioperative management
1. **Cardiovascular system**
   a. Burn patients require aggressive fluid resuscitation during the first 24-48 hours.
   b. **Fluid replacement protocols**
      (1) Parkland formula: 4.0 cc of Ringer's lactate per kg per %TBSA per 24 hours.
      (2) Half the calculated fluid deficit is administered during the first 8 hours after the burn injury, and the remainder is given over the next 16 hours. Daily maintenance fluid requirements should be given concurrently.
   c. Early cardiovascular effects include decreased cardiac output, decreased arterial blood pressure, and increased capillary permeability.

2. **Respiratory system**
   a. Thermal injury of the face and upper airway are common. Inhalational injury should be suspected in the presence of facial or intraoral burns, singed nasal hairs, a brassy cough, carbonaceous sputum, and wheezing. Before airway edema occurs, endotracheal intubation should be performed.
   b. Carbon monoxide poisoning is defined as greater than 20% carboxyhemoglobin in the blood. Tissue hypoxia ensues.
   c. Manifestations of carbon monoxide poisoning include irritability, headache, nausea/vomiting, visual disturbances, seizures, coma, or death.
   d. Pulse oximetry overestimates the oxyhemoglobin saturation in the presence of carboxyhemoglobin because the absorption spectrum is similar. The classic cherry red color of the skin is a sign of high concentrations of carbon monoxide.

C. Anesthetic considerations
1. Succinylcholine is contraindicated 24 hours to 2 years after major burns because it can produce profound hyperkalemia and cardiac arrest.
2. Nondepolarizing muscle relaxants are used when muscle relaxation is required. Burn patients require higher than normal doses of nondepolarizing muscle relaxants.
3. Burn patients may have increased narcotic requirements because of tolerance and increases in the apparent volume of distribution.

V. Cardiac tamponade
A. Manifestations
1. Dyspnea, orthopnea, tachycardia. Beck's triad consists of hypotension, distant heart sounds, distention of jugular veins.
2. Paradoxical pulse (>10 mmHg decline in BP during inspiration).
3. The principle hemodynamic feature is a decrease in cardiac output from a reduced stroke volume with an increase in central venous pressure. Equalization of diastolic pressures occur throughout the heart. Impairment of both diastolic filling and atrial emptying abolishes the 'y' descent; the 'x' descent is normal.
4. EKG: ST segment changes, electrical alternans.
5. CXR: silhouette normal or slightly enlarged.
6. Transesophageal echo is the best diagnostic tool.

B. Anesthetic considerations
1. Maintain filling pressures (to maximize stroke volume). Support myocardial contractility with inotropic support if necessary. Avoid bradycardia.
2. Avoid positive pressure ventilation because increased intrathoracic pressure will impede venous return and exacerbate underfilling of the cardiac chambers.
3. Pre-induction monitors: Standard monitors plus arterial line and central venous line (and pulmonary artery catheter if needed).
4. Hemodynamically unstable patients should be managed with pericardiocentesis (under local anesthesia) prior to induction (the removal of even a small amount of fluid can improve cardiac performance).
5. Induction: ketamine is the drug of choice, however, ketamine depresses myocardial contractility and may precipitate hemodynamic deterioration when used in the presence of hypovolemia and maximal sympathetic outflow.

Ophthalmologic Surgery

I. Physiology of intraocular pressure
   A. Normal intraocular pressure is maintained between 10 and 20 mmHg.
   B. Aqueous humor is formed at a rate of 2 microliters/min. Two thirds is secreted by the ciliary body via an active sodium-pump mechanism. One third is produced by passive ultrafiltration through vessels on the anterior iris. Fluid ultimately drains through the Canal of Schlemm.
   C. Intraocular pressure is controlled primarily by regulation of the outflow resistance at the trabecular meshwork. Acute changes in choroidal blood volume can produce rapid increases in intraocular pressure. Hypercapnia can lead to choroidal congestion and increased intraocular pressure. The increases in venous pressure associated with coughing, straining, or vomiting can raise IOP to 30 to 40 mmHg. Similar increases can be seen at intubation. Intraocular pressure can also be increased by extrinsic compression of the globe. The force of the eyelid in a normal blink may cause an increase of 10 mmHg; a forceful lid squeeze can increase IOP to over 50 mmHg A poorly placed anesthesia mask could increase IOP to the point of zero blood flow.
   D. Choroidal blood flow is normally autoregulated.

II. Oculocardiac reflex
   A. Traction on extraocular muscles or pressure on the globe can elicit cardiac dysrhythmias ranging from bradycardia and ventricular ectopy to sinus arrest or ventricular fibrillation.
   B. The reflex is trigeminovagal. The afferent limb is from orbital contents to the ciliary ganglion to the ophthalmic division of the trigeminal nerve to the sensory nucleus of the trigeminal nerve near the fourth ventricle. The efferent limb is via the vagus nerve. The reflex fatigues with repeated traction on the extraocular muscles.
   C. Prevention
      1. Retrobulbar block is not uniformly effective in preventing the reflex (retrobulbar block may elicit the oculocardiac reflex).
      2. Anticholinergic medication can be effective, however caution must be used in the elderly.
      3. Deepen anesthesia.
      4. Factors associated with increased susceptibility to the development of ocularcardiac reflex are anxiety, hypoxia, hypercarbia, and light anesthesia.
   C. Treatment
      1. Request the surgeon to stop manipulation.
      2. Assess adequate ventilation, oxygenation, and depth of anesthesia.
      3. If severe or persistent bradycardia, give atropine (7-10 mcg/kg).
      4. In recurrent episodes, infiltration of the rectus muscles with local anesthetics.

III. Intraocular gas expansion
   A. A gas bubble may be injected into the posterior chamber during vitreous surgery to flatten a detached retina.
   B. The air bubble is absorbed within 5 days by gradual diffusion.
   C. Sulfur hexafluoride, an inert gas that is less soluble in blood than nitrogen, provides a longer duration (up to 10 days) in comparison with an air bubble.
   D. Nitrous oxide should be discontinued at least 15 minutes prior to the

injection of air or sulfur hexafluoride. Nitrous oxide should be avoided until the bubble is absorbed (5 days for air and 10 days for sulfur hexafluoride injection).

IV. Anesthetic drugs

A. Most anesthetic drugs either lower or have no effect on intraocular pressure. An exception is ketamine, and possibly etomidate.

B. Ketamine effects are controversial, but is generally felt to moderately increase intraocular pressure. Ketamine increases choroidal blood flow, increases nystagmus, and increases extraocular muscle tone via blepharospasm.

C. Etomidate, which is associated with a high incidence of myoclonus (10-60%), may increase intraocular pressure.

D. Succinylcholine can cause a 5-10 mmHg increase in intraocular pressure for 5-10 minutes. Succinylcholine can potentially increase intraocular pressure by dilating choroidal blood vessels and increases in extraocular muscle tone. Pretreatment with a defasiculating dose of a nondepolarizing muscle relaxant does not reliably eliminate the effect of succinylcholine on intraocular pressure. Nondepolarizing muscle relaxants do not increase intraocular pressure.

V. Systemic effects of ophthalmic drugs

A. Anticholinesterases (echothiophate, phospholine iodide): Systemic absorption leads to inhibition of plasma cholinesterase which may lead to prolongation of succinylcholine's duration of action. Takes 3 weeks for pseudocholinesterase levels to return to 50% of normal. The metabolism of mivacurium and ester-type local anesthetics may also be affected.

B. Cholinergics (pilocarpine, acetylcholine): Used to induce miosis; toxicity may manifest in bradycardia or acute bronchospasm.

C. Anticholinergics (atropine, scopolamine): Used to cause mydriasis; systemic absorption may lead to tachycardia, dry skin, fever, and agitation.

D. Beta-blockers (timolol maleate): Systemic absorption may cause beta-blockade (bradycardia, bronchospasm, or exacerbation of congestive heart failure). Betaxolol seems to be oculo-specific with minimal side effects.

E. Carbonic anhydrase inhibitors (acetazolamide, Diamox): Used to decrease aqueous production; induces an alkaline diuresis. Side effects include diuresis and hypokalemic metabolic acidosis.

VI. Retrobulbar blockade

A. Technique: Local anesthetic is injected behind the eye into the cone formed by the extraocular muscles. Lidocaine and bupivacaine are the most commonly used local anesthetics. Hyaluronidase, a hydrolyzer of connective tissue polysaccharides, is commonly added to enhance the spread of local anesthetic.

B. Complications: Retrobulbar hemorrhage, globe perforation, optic nerve atrophy, convulsions, oculocardiac reflex, loss of consciousness, and respiratory arrest.

C. Post-retrobulbar apnea syndrome: Due to injection of local anesthetic into the optic nerve sheath with spread into the cerebrospinal fluid. Apnea typically occurs within 20 minutes and may last 15-60 minutes. Adequacy of ventilation must be constantly monitored in patients with retrobulbar blocks.

D. Facial nerve block prevents squinting of the eyelid. Major complications include subcutaneous hemorrhage.

Transurethral Resection of the Prostate

I. **Complications**
   A. Intravascular absorption of irrigating fluid: The amount of solution absorbed depends on the hydrostatic pressure of the irrigating fluid, the duration of time sinuses are exposed to irrigating fluid (10 to 30 mL of irrigating fluid is absorbed per minute), and the number and sizes of the venous sinuses opened during resection. Absorption of the irrigating fluid can result in fluid overload, serum hypoosmolality, hyponatremia, hyperglycemia, hyperammonemia, hemolysis.
   B. Autotransfusion secondary to lithotomy position. Hypothermia may occur. Bacteremia has an incidence of 10% in patients with sterile urine and an incidence of 50% in patients with infected urine.
   C. Blood loss: Related to vascularity of the prostate gland, technique, weight of the prostate resected, length of the operation. Perforation of bladder or urethra.
   D. Transient blindness: Attributed to absorption of glycine and its metabolic byproduct, ammonia, acting as an inhibitory neurotransmitter in the retina.
   E. CNS toxicity: Result of oxidative biotransformation of glycine to ammonia.
   F. CNS symptoms, including apprehension, irritability, confusion, headache, seizures, transient blindness, and coma, have all been attributed to hyponatremia and hyposmolarity.

II. **Management of TURP Syndrome and hyponatremia**
   A. Obtain serum sodium and arterial blood gas.
   B. Serum sodium >120 mEq/L: Obtain hemostasis; terminate transurethral surgery; oxygen by mask or nasal cannula; fluid restriction; brisk diuresis with loop diuretics.
   C. Serum sodium <120 mEq/L: Obtain hemostasis; terminate transurethral surgery; oxygen by mask or nasal cannula; fluid restriction; loop diuretics; consider hypertonic saline (eg, 3% or 5% saline) infused at a rate which does not exceed 100 mL/hr. Allow sodium to rise by 0.5-2.0 mEq/l/hr; stop hypertonic saline and loop diuretics once sodium is 120-130 mEq/l.

Electroconvulsive Therapy

I. **Cardiovascular response**. Initial parasympathetic outflow may result in bradycardia. The parasympathetic response is followed by a sympathetic outflow, which produces hypertension and tachycardia, usually lasting 5-10 minutes.

II. **Anesthetic Management**
   A. Methohexital 0.5-1.0 mg/kg and succinylcholine 0.25-0.5 mg/kg.
   B. Place blood pressure cuff on the opposite arm of the IV and inflate prior to the administration of succinylcholine to allow for motor expression of the seizure.
   C. Induced seizures should last longer than 25 seconds and should be terminated if they last longer than 3 minutes.

III. **Pain control**
   A. Moderate to severe postoperative pain in the PACU can be managed with parenteral opioids.
      1. Meperidine 25-50 mg (0.25-0.5 mg/kg in children).
      2. Morphine 2-4 mg (0.025-0.05 mg/kg in children).

3. Fentanyl 12.5-50 mcg IV.
   B. Nonsteroidal antiinflammatory drugs are an effective complement to opioids. Ketorolac 30 mg IV followed by 15 mg q6-8 hrs.

Laparoscopic Surgery

I. **Pulmonary effects.** Laparoscopy creates of a pneumoperitoneum with pressurized CO_2 (up to a pressure of 30 cm H_2O). The resulting increase in intra-abdominal pressure displaces the diaphragm cephalad, causing a decrease in lung compliance and an increase in peak inspiratory pressure. Atelectasis, diminished functional residual capacity, ventilation/perfusion mismatch, and pulmonary shunting contribute to a decrease in arterial oxygenation. The high solubility of CO_2 increases systemic absorption which can lead to increased arterial CO_2 levels.

II. **Cardiac effects.** Moderate insufflation can increase effective cardiac filling because blood tends to be forced out of the abdomen and into the chest. Higher insufflation pressures (greater than 25 cm H_2O), however, tends to collapse the major abdominal veins which compromises venous return and leads to a drop in preload and cardiac output in some patients. Hypercarbia may stimulate the sympathetic nervous system and thus increase blood pressure, heart rate, and risk of dysrhythmias.

III. **Management of anesthesia**
   A. **Patient position.** Trendelenburg is often associated with a decrease in FRC, VC, TLV, and pulmonary compliance.
   B. **Anesthetic technique.** General anesthesia with endotracheal intubation is the preferred technique.
   C. **Complications.** Hemorrhage, peritonitis, subcutaneous emphysemas pneumomediastinum, pneumothorax, and venous air embolism. Vagal stimulation during trocar insertion, peritoneal insufflation, or manipulation of viscera can result in bradycardia and sinus arrest.

Myasthenia Gravis

I. Myasthenia gravis is characterized by weakness and easy fatigability of skeletal muscle. The weakness is thought to be due to autoimmune destruction or inactivation of postsynaptic acetylcholine receptors at the neuromuscular junction. Muscle strength characteristically improves with rest but deteriorates rapidly with repeated effort.

II. **Osserman classification**
   A. Type I: Involvement of extraocular muscles only.
   B. Type IIa: Mild skeletal muscle weakness, spares muscles of respiration.
   C. Type IIb: More severe skeletal muscle weakness with bulbar involvement.
   D. Type III: Acute onset, rapid deterioration, severe bulbar and skeletal muscle involvement.
   E. Type IV: Late, severe involvement of bulbar and skeletal muscle.

III. **Treatment of Myasthenia Gravis**
   A. Treatment consists of anticholinesterase drugs, immunosuppressants, glucocorticoids, plasmapheresis, and thymectomy.
   B. Anticholinesterase drugs (usually pyridostigmine) inhibit the breakdown of acetylcholine by tissue cholinesterase, increasing the amount of

acetylcholine at the neuromuscular junction.
- C. Cholinergic crisis is characterized by increased weakness and excessive muscarinic effect, including salivation, diarrhea, miosis, and bradycardia.
- D. Edrophonium test: used to differentiate a cholinergic crisis form a myasthenic crisis. Increased weakness after up to 10 mg of intravenous edrophonium is indicative of cholinergic crisis, whereas increasing strength implies myasthenic crisis.

IV. **Pre-op predictors** for post-op ventilation (after transsternal thymectomy).
- A. Duration of disease greater than 6 years.
- B. Presence of COPD or other lung disease unrelated to myasthenia.
- C. Pyridostigmine dose greater than 750 mg/day.
- D. Preoperative FVC less than 2.9 liters.

V. **Anesthetic concerns.** Muscle relaxants should be avoided. The response to succinylcholine is unpredictable. Patients may manifest a relative resistance, a prolonged effect, or an unusual response (phase II block).

Myasthenic Syndrome

I. Myasthenic syndrome, also called Eaton-Lambert syndrome, is a paraneoplastic syndrome characterized by proximal muscle weakness, which typically affects the lower extremities. Myasthenic syndrome is usually associated with small-cell carcinoma of the lung. In contrast to myasthenia gravis, the muscle weakness improves with repeated effort and is unaffected by anticholinesterase drugs.

II. Patients with the myasthenic syndrome are very sensitive to both depolarizing and nondepolarizing muscle relaxants.

Anesthesia for Organ Harvest

I. **The donor**
- A. Brain death should be pronounced prior to going to the OR.
- B. **Clinical criteria for brain death**
    1. Cerebral unresponsiveness, irreversible coma.
    2. Brain stem unresponsiveness.
    3. Fixed and dilated pupils, doll's eyes, negative caloric test, absent corneal reflex.
    4. Absent gag and cough reflex, apnea (no respiratory efforts with $PaCO_2$ greater than 60 mmHg).
    5. No posturing (spinal reflexes may be present).
- C. **Ancillary tests**
    1. Isoelectric electroencephalogram.
    2. Absent cerebral blood flow by intracranial angiography or nuclear brain scan.
    3. Body temperature less than 95 degrees F.
    4. Absence of drug intoxication or neuromuscular blocking agents.
    5. Corrected metabolic abnormalities.

II. **Donor management**
- A. Overall goals are restoration and maintenance of hemodynamic and

vascular stability. Hemodynamics should be maintained as follows:
1. Systolic blood pressure greater than 100 mmHg.
2. Central venous pressure 10-12 mmHg.
3. Urine output greater than 100 cc/hour.
4. P_aO_2 greater than 100 mmHg.

B. Physiologic changes associated with brain death

1. Cardiovascular instability is a common feature, secondary to loss of neurologic control of the myocardium and vascular tree. Fluid resuscitation should be used to keep systolic blood pressure greater than 100 mmHg and mean arterial pressure greater than 70 mmHg.
2. Central diabetes insipidus may occur from hypothalamic failure resulting in extreme salt and water wasting from the kidneys. Massive loss of fluid and electrolytes that may occur. Aqueous Pitressin should be administered in doses of 10 units intravenously every 4 hours to bring urine output down to 150-200 cc per hour.
3. Loss of thermoregulatory control. After brain death, body temperature drifts downward to core temperature.
4. Neurogenic pulmonary edema may be present.
5. Coagulopathy: the release of tissue fibrinolytic agent from a necrotic brain may initiates coagulopathy.
6. Hypoxia: pulmonary insufficiency secondary to trauma and/or shock should be treated with mechanical ventilation, positive end-expiratory pressure (PEEP), and inspired oxygen fraction sufficient to maintain adequate peripheral oxygen delivery.
7. Overall hypovolemia is the most important variable affecting donor organ perfusion. Ringer's lactate should be infused to establish a central venous pressure of 10-12 mmHg. Hematocrit should be maintained about 30%.
8. Anesthesia is not needed in the brain dead patient. However, significant hemodynamic responses to surgical stimuli commonly occur in the brain-dead donor during organ harvesting. These responses may reflect some residual lower medullary function (visceral and somatic reflexes). Movement secondary to spinal reflex action should be controlled. Patients are routinely declared dead prior to going to the operating room.

Postanesthesia Care Unit

I. **Hemodynamic complications**
   A. **Hypotension**
      1. **Differential diagnosis.** Inadequate venous return (hypovolemia), decreased vascular tone (neuroaxial anesthesia, sepsis), decreased inotropy (myocardial ischemia, dysrhythmias), spurious (wide cuff), and pulmonary edema (excess fluids).
      2. **Treatment.** Fluid challenge. Pharmacologic treatment includes inotropic agents (dopamine, dobutamine, epinephrine) and alpha receptor agonists (phenylephrine, epinephrine).
   B. **Hypertension**
      1. **Differential diagnosis.** Most common cause is preexistent hypertension. Other etiologies include pain, bladder distention, fluid overload, hypoxemia, spurious (cuff too narrow), increased intracranial pressure, and vasopressors.
      2. **Treatment.** Resuming chronic antihypertensive therapy, nitroprusside, beta blockers (labetalol 5-10 mg IV, esmolol 10-100 mg IV) or calcium channel blockers (nifedipine 5-10 mg SL, verapamil 2.5-5 mg IV).
   C. **Dysrhythmias**
      1. Possible etiologies of perioperative dysrhythmias include increased sympathetic outflow, hypoxemia, hypercarbia, electrolyte and acid-base imbalances, myocardial ischemia, increased ICP, drug toxicity, and malignant hyperthermia.
      2. Supplemental oxygen should be given while the etiology is being investigated.
   D. **Myocardial ischemia and infarction**
      1. Common causes include hypoxemia, anemia, tachycardia, hypotension, and hypertension.
      2. Treatment. Supplemental oxygen and obtain 12 lead EKG.

II. **Respiratory complications**
   A. **Respiratory problems** are the most frequently encountered complications in the PACU, with the majority related to airway obstruction, hypoventilation, or hypoxemia.
   B. **Hypoxemia**
      1. Causes of hypoxemia include atelectasis, hypoventilation, diffusion hypoxia, upper airway obstruction, bronchospasm, aspiration of gastric contents, pulmonary edema, pneumothorax and pulmonary embolism.
      2. Clinically, hypoxia may also be suspected from restlessness, tachycardia, or cardiac irritability. Obtundation, bradycardia, hypotension, and cardiac arrest are late signs.
      3. Increased intrapulmonary shunting relative to closing capacity is the most common of hypoxemia following general anesthesia.
      4. Treatment. Oxygen therapy with or without positive airway pressure. Additional treatment should be directed at the underlying cause.
   C. **Hypoventilation**
      1. Etiologies include decreased ventilatory drive, pulmonary, and respiratory muscle insufficiency (preexistent respiratory disease, inadequate reversal of neuromuscular blockade, inadequate analgesia, and bronchospasm).
      2. Hypoventilation in the PACU is most commonly caused by residual depressant effects of anesthetic agents on respiratory drive.

3. Treatment should be directed at the underlying cause. Marked hypoventilation may require controlled ventilation until contributory factors are identified and corrected.

D. Upper airway obstruction
1. Etiologies include incomplete anesthetic recovery, laryngospasm, airway edema, wound hematoma, and vocal cord paralysis. Airway obstruction in unconscious patients is most commonly due to the tongue falling back against the posterior pharynx.
2. Patients with airway obstruction should receive supplemental oxygen while corrective measures are undertaken. Jaw thrust, head-tilt, oral or nasal airways often alleviate the problem.

E. Laryngospasm
1. Laryngospasm is a forceful involuntary spasm of the laryngeal musculature caused by sensory stimulation of the superior laryngeal nerve. Triggering stimuli include pharyngeal secretions or extubating in stage 2. The large negative intrathoracic pressures generated by the struggling patient in laryngospasm can cause pulmonary edema.
2. Treatment. initial treatment includes 100% oxygen, anterior mandibular displacement, and gentle CPAP (may be applied by face mask). If laryngospasm persists and hypoxia develops, succinylcholine (0.25-1.0 mg/kg; 10-20 mg) should be given in order to paralyze the laryngeal muscles and allow controlled ventilation.
3. Treatment of glottic edema and subglottic edema. Administer warm, humidified oxygen by mask, inhalation of racemic epinephrine 2.25% (0.5-1 mL in 2 mL NS), repeated every 20 minutes, dexamethasone 0.1-0.5 mg/kg IV. Reintubation with a smaller tube may be helpful.

III. Shivering
A. Shivering can occur secondary to hypothermia or the effects of anesthetic agents (most often volatile anesthetics).
B. Shivering should be treated with warming measures. Small doses of meperidine (12.5-25 mg) IV and can dramatically reduce shivering.

IV. Neurologic complications
A. Delayed awakening. The most frequent cause of a delayed awakening is the persistent effect of anesthesia or sedation. Other causes include recurarization, severe hypothermia, hypoglycemia, and neurologic disorders.

B. Emergence delirium is characterized by excitement, alternating with lethargy, disorientation, and inappropriate behavior. Treatment includes haloperidol, titrated in 1-2 mg IV increments. Benzodiazepines may be added if agitation is severe. Physostigmine (0.5-2.0 mg IV) may reverse anticholinergic delirium.

V. Nausea/vomiting
A. Risk factors
1. **Patient factors.** Younger age, female, obesity, anxiety, gastroparesis, history of postoperative nausea/vomiting or motion sickness.
2. **Surgical procedures.** Gynecological, abdominal, ENT, ophthalmic, plastic surgery.

B. Anesthetic factors. Premedicants (morphine and other opioid compounds), anesthetics agents (nitrous oxide, inhalational agents, etomidate, methohexital, balanced techniques), anticholinesterase reversal agents, gastric distention, longer duration of anesthesia.

C. Postoperative factors. Pain, dizziness, movement after surgery, premature oral intake, opioid administration.

D. Treatment
1. Droperidol 0.625-1.25 mg IV.
2. Metoclopramide 10 mg.
3. Prochlorperazine 5-10 mg IV.
4. Promethazine 12.5-25 mg IV.

VI. Pain control
A. Moderate to severe postoperative pain in the PACU can be managed with parenteral opioids.
1. Meperidine 25-50 mg (0.25-0.5 mg/kg in children).
2. Morphine 2-4 mg (0.025-0.05 mg/kg in children).
3. Fentanyl 12.5-50 mcg IV.

B. Nonsteroidal anti-inflammatory drugs are an effective complement to opioids. Ketorolac 30 mg IV followed by 15 mg q6-8 hrs.
C. Patient-controlled and continuous epidural analgesia should be started in the PACU.

VII. Discharge criteria
A. All patients must be evaluated by an anesthesiologist prior to discharge from the PACU. Before discharge, patients should have been observed for respiratory depression for at least 30 minutes after the last dose of parenteral narcotic.
B. Patients receiving regional anesthesia should show signs of resolution of both sensory and motor blockade.
C. Other minimum discharge criteria for patients include stable vital signs, alert and oriented (or to baseline), able to maintain adequate oxygen saturation, free of nausea/vomiting, absence of bleeding, adequate urine output, adequate pain control, stabilization or resolution of any problems, and movement of extremity following regional anesthesia.

Malignant Hyperthermia

I. Definition.
Malignant hyperthermia is a fulminant skeletal muscle hypermetabolic syndrome occurring in genetically susceptible patients after exposure to an anesthetic triggering agent. Triggering anesthetics include halothane, enflurane, isoflurane, desflurane, sevoflurane, and succinylcholine.

II. Etiology.
The gene for malignant hyperthermia is the genetic coding site for the calcium release channel of skeletal muscle sarcoplasmic reticulum (ryanodine receptor). The syndrome is caused by a reduction in the reuptake of calcium by the sarcoplasmic reticulum necessary for termination of muscle contraction, resulting in a sustained muscle contraction.

III. Clinical findings
A. Signs of onset. tachycardia, tachypnea, hypercarbia (increased end-tidal CO_2 is the most sensitive clinical sign).
B. Early signs. Tachycardia, tachypnea, unstable blood pressure, arrhythmias, cyanosis, mottling, sweating, rapid temperature increase, and cola-colored urine.
C. Late (6-24 hours) signs. Pyrexia, skeletal muscle swelling, left heart failure, renal failure, DIC, hepatic failure.
D. Muscle rigidity in the presence of neuromuscular blockade. Masseter spasm after giving succinylcholine is associated with malignant hyperthermia.

Malignant Hyperthermia

- **E.** The presence of a large difference between mixed venous and arterial carbon dioxide tensions confirms the diagnosis of malignant hyperthermia.
- **F.** Laboratory. Respiratory and metabolic acidosis, hypoxemia, increased serum levels of potassium, calcium, myoglobin, CPK, and myoglobinuria.

IV. Incidence and mortality
- **A.** Children. Approx 1:12,000 general anesthetics.
- **B.** Adults. Approx 1:40,000 general anesthetics when succinylcholine is used; approx 1:220,000 general anesthetics when agents other than succinylcholine are used.
- **C.** Familial autosomal dominant transmission with variable penetrance.
- **D.** Mortality. 10% overall; up to 70% without dantrolene therapy. Early therapy reduces mortality for less than 5%.

V. Anesthesia for malignant hyperthermia susceptible patients
- **A.** Malignant hyperthermia may be triggered in susceptible patients who have had previous uneventful responses to triggering agents.
- **B.** Pretreatment with dantrolene is generally not recommended.
- **C.** The anesthesia machine should be prepared by flushing the circuit with ten liters per minute of oxygen for 20 minutes. Changing the fresh gas hose will hasten the reduction of the concentration of inhalation agents. Fresh carbon dioxide absorbent and fresh delivery tubing are also recommended.

VI. Malignant hyperthermia treatment protocol
- **A.** Stop triggering anesthetic agents immediately, conclude surgery as soon as possible. Continue with safe agents if surgery cannot be stopped.
- **B.** Hyperventilate. 100% oxygen at high flows. Use new circuit and soda lime.
- **C.** Administer dantrolene 2.5 mg/kg IV. Continue until all signs normalize (up to 10 mg/kg).
- **D.** Correct metabolic acidosis. Administer sodium bicarbonate, 1-2 mEq/kg IV guided by arterial pH and pCO_2. Follow with ABG. Hyperkalemia: Correct with bicarbonate or with glucose, 25-50 gm IV, and regular insulin, 10-20 u.
- **E. Actively cool patient**
    1. Iced IV NS (not ringer's lactate) 15 mL/kg every 10 minutes times three if needed.
    2. Lavage stomach, bladder, rectum, peritoneal and thoracic cavities with iced NS.
    3. Surface cool with ice and hypothermia blanket.
- **F.** Maintain urine output >1-2 mL/kg/hr. If needed, mannitol 0.25 g/kg IV or furosemide 1 mg/kg IV (up to 4 times).
- **G.** Labs. PT, PTT, platelets, urine myoglobin, ABG, K, Ca, lactate, CPK.
- **H.** Consider invasive monitoring of arterial blood pressure and central venous pressure.
- **I.** Postoperatively. Continue dantrolene 1 mg/kg IV q6 hours x 72 hrs to prevent recurrence. Observe in ICU until stable for 24-48 hrs. Calcium channel blockers should not be given when dantrolene is administered because hyperkalemia and myocardial depression may occur.

Allergic Drug Reactions

I. Anaphylaxis
A. Anaphylaxis is an allergic reaction which is mediated by an antigen-antibody reaction (type I hypersensitivity reaction). This reaction is initiated by antigen binding to immunoglobulin E (IgE) antibodies on the surface of mast cells and basophils, causing the release of chemical mediators, including, leukotrienes, histamine, prostaglandins, kinins, and platelet-activating factor.

B. **Clinical manifestations of anaphylaxis**
1. **Cardiovascular.** Hypotension, tachycardia, dysrhythmias.
2. **Pulmonary.** Bronchospasm, cough, dyspnea, pulmonary edema, laryngeal edema, hypoxemia.
3. **Dermatologic.** Urticaria, facial edema, pruritus.

II. Anaphylactoid reactions
A. Anaphylactoid reactions resemble anaphylaxis but are not mediated by IgE and do not require prior sensitization to an antigen.

B. Although the mechanisms differ, anaphylactic and anaphylactoid reactions can be clinically indistinguishable and equally life-threatening.

III. Treatment of anaphylactic and anaphylactoid reactions
A. **Initial therapy**
1. Discontinue drug administration and all anesthetic agents.
2. Administer 100% oxygen.
3. Intravenous fluids (1-5 liters of LR).
4. Epinephrine (10-100 mcg IV bolus for hypotension; 0.1-0.5 mg IV for cardiovascular collapse).

B. **Secondary treatment**
1. Benadryl 0.5-1 mg/kg or 50-75 mg IV.
2. Epinephrine 2-4. mcg/min, norepinephrine 2-4 mcg/min, titrated to effect.
3. Aminophylline 5-6 mg/kg IV over 20 minutes with persistent bronchospasm.
4. 1-2 grams methylprednisolone or 0.25-1 gram hydrocortisone.
5. Sodium bicarbonate (0.5-1 mEq/kg with persistent hypotension or acidosis).
6. Airway evaluation (prior to extubation).

Venous Air Embolism

I. General information
A. Air can be entrained into a vein whenever there is an open vein and a negative intravenous pressure relative to atmospheric pressure. This can occur any time the surgical field is above right atrial level (neurosurgical procedures and operations involving the neck, thorax, abdomen, pelvis, open heart, liver and vena cava laceration repairs, total hip replacement).

B. Incidence is highest during sitting craniotomies (20-40%).

II. Diagnosis
A. Transesophageal echocardiography (TEE) is the most sensitive. Sensitivity = 0.015 mL of air/kg/min.

B. Doppler. Sensitivity equals 0.02 mL of air/kg/min.

C. Decreased PaO_2, TcO_2, and increased ETN_2 (most specific) normally occur before one sees a sudden decrease in $ETCO_2$ and/or an increase in CVP.
D. During controlled ventilation of the lungs, sudden attempts by the patient to initiate a spontaneous breath (gasp reflex) may be the first indication of venous air embolism.
E. Hypotension, tachycardia, cardiac dysrhythmias and cyanosis are late signs of a venous air embolism.
F. Consequences depend of the volume and rate of air entry.
  1. CVP increases 0.4 mL of air/kg/min.
  2. Heart rate increases at 0.42 mL of air/kg/min.
  3. EKG changes occur at 0.6 mL of air/kg/min.
  4. Blood pressure decreases at 0.69 mL of air/kg/min.
  5. A mill wheel murmur is heard at 2.0 mL of air/kg/min.
  6. Embolism of greater than 2.0 mL of air/kg/min is potentially lethal.

III. Treatment
A. Notify surgeon to flood surgical field with saline or pack and apply bone wax to the skull edges until the entry site identified.
B. Place the patient in the left lateral decubitus position with a slight head-down tilt in an attempt to dislodge a possible air lock.
C. Nitrous oxide should be discontinued and 100% oxygen given.
D. The central venous catheter should be aspirated in an attempt to retrieve the entrained air.
E. Support cardiovascular system with volume, inotropes, and/or vasopressors.
F. Increase venous pressure with bilateral jugular vein compression.

Latex Allergy

I. Risk factors for latex allergy
A. Chronic exposure to latex and a history of atopy increases the risk of sensitization. Patients undergoing frequent procedures with latex items (eg, repeated urinary bladder catheterization) are at higher risk.
B. Patients with neural tube defects (meningomyelocele, spina bifida) and those with congenital abnormalities of the genitourinary tract are at higher risk.

II. Pathophysiology.
Most reactions involve a direct IgE-mediated immune response to polypeptides in natural latex. Some cases of contact dermatitis may be due to a type four hypersensitivity reaction to chemicals introduced in the manufacturing process.

III. Preoperative evaluation
A. **History** in patients at risk, particularly those with co-existing atopy and/or multiple allergies, should include history of balloon or glove intolerance and allergies to medical products used in chronic care (eg, catheters). Elective patients in whom latex allergy is suspected should be referred to an allergist.
B. **Diagnostic tests.** Routine diagnostic testing in the at-risk population is not recommended (only those with a positive history). Available tests include the following:
  1. Skin-prick test: less sensitive than intradermal test but more sensitive than RAST.

158 Latex Allergy

   2. Radioallergosorbent test (RAST). An in-vitro test for IgE antibodies in the patient's serum.
   3. Pre-operative medications. Routine preoperative H_1 and H_2 blockers and steroids is no longer recommended.
   4. Scheduling. since latex is an aeroallergen and present in the operating room air for at least an hour after the use of latex gloves, whenever possible your patient should be scheduled as the first case of the day.

IV. Anesthesia equipment
   A. Common anesthesia equipment that contain latex include gloves, tourniquets, endotracheal tube, ventilator bellows, intravenous injection ports, blood pressure cuffs, and face masks.
   B. Non-latex supplies that are commonly required include glass syringes, drugs in glass in ampules, IV tubing without latex injection ports, neoprene gloves, ambu bag with silicone valves, and neoprene bellows for the Ohmeda ventilator.
   C. The most important precaution is the use of non-latex gloves.
   D. Misc equipment. Sleeve on the fibreoptic bronchoscope is non-latex, esophageal stethoscope is non-latex, cuff on the LMA airway is non-latex (silicon).

V. Preoperative preparation
   A. Check latex allergy cart for supplies. Call pharmacy and order all drugs that may be needed (dispensed in glass syringe).
   B. Notify O.R. nurses on service. No latex gloves or latex products should come into contact with the patient. Neoprene (non-latex) gloves need to be obtained.

VI. Anesthesia setup and care
   A. Set up a regular circuit on the anesthesia machine, and use a neoprene reservoir bag. Use plastic masks (adult or pediatric).
   B. Draw up drugs in glass syringes from glass ampules. In an emergency, the rubber stoppers can be removed, and drug can be drawn up in a glass syringe.
   C. IV infusion setup with two three way stopcocks and no injection ports. (Alternatively tape all injection ports over and do not use).
   D. Use Webril under the rubber tourniquet for IV placement. Teflon catheters can be used safely (eg, Angiocath). If BP cuff is rubber, use Webril under it.
   E. Latex allergy should not alter the choice of anesthetic technique. There are no drugs that are specifically contraindicated.

VII. Diagnosis of latex anaphylaxis
   A. Anaphylaxis has been reported even in patients pre-treated with H_1, H_2 blockers and steroids and managed in a latex-free environment.
   B. Onset is generally 20 - 60 minutes after exposure to the antigen.
   C. Anaphylaxis presents with the clinical triad of hypotension (most common sign), rash, and bronchospasm.
   D. Serum mast cell tryptase levels are high during an episode and up to 4 hours after. This test will help confirm the diagnosis of anaphylaxis, but it will not identify latex as the antigen.

VIII. Treatment of latex anaphylaxis
   A. Treatment of latex anaphylaxis does not differ from the treatment of other forms of anaphylactic reaction.
   B. Primary treatment
   1. Stop administration of latex. Administer 100% oxygen.

2. Restore intravascular volume (2-4 L of crystalloid).
3. Epinephrine. Start with a dose of 10 mcg, or 0.1 mcg/kg and escalate rapidly to higher doses depending on the response.

C. Secondary treatment
1. Corticosteroids (0.25-1 g hydrocortisone or 1-2 g methylprednisolone).
2. Diphenhydramine 50-75 mg IV.
3. Aminophylline (5-6 mg/kg over 20 minutes for persistent bronchospasm).

References

1. Barash PG, Cullen BF, Stoelting RK (eds): Clinical Anesthesia. JB Lippincott, Philadelphia, 1992.
2. Blitt, CD (ed): Monitoring in Anesthesia and Critical Care Medicine. Second edition. Churchill Livingstone, New York, 1990.
3. Cucchiara RF, Michenfelder, JD: Clinical Neuroanesthesia. Churchill Livingstone, New York, 1990.
4. DiNardo JA, Schwartz MJ: Anesthesia for Cardiac Surgery. Appleton and Lange, Connecticut, 1990.
5. Emergency Cardiac Care Committee and Subcommittees, American Heart Association. Guidelines for Cardiopulmonary Resuscitation and Emergency Cardiac Care. JAMA. 1992;268.
6. Guyton A: Textbook of Medical Physiology. Seventh edition. WB Saunders, Philadelphia, 1986.
7. Kaplan JA (ed): Cardiac Anesthesia. Third edition. WB Saunders, Philadephia, 1993.
8. Miller RD (ed): Anesthesia. Third edition. Churchill Livingstone, New York, 1990.
9. Nunn JF: Applied Respiratory Physiology. Third edition. Butterworth, London, 1987.
10. Shnider SM, Levinson, G: Anesthesia for Obstetrics. Third edition. Williams and Wilkins, Maryland, 1993.
11. Stoelting, RK: Pharmacology and Physiology in Aesthetic Practice. JB Lippincott, Philadelphia, 1987.
12. Stoelting RK, Dierdorf SF, McCammon RC: Anesthesia and Co-Existing Disease. Second edition. Churchill Livingstone, New York, 1988.
13. Stoelting RK, Miller RD: Basics of Anesthesia. Second edition. Churchill Livingstone, New York, 1989.
14. Rogers MC (ed): Current Practice in Anesthesiology. Second edition. Mosby Year Book, Missouri, 1992.
15. Tarhan, S et al: Myocardial infarction after general anesthesia. JAMA 220:1451-1454, 1972.

Index

A-a gradient 72
Abruptio placentae 132
Acetaminophen 140
Acetohexamide 21
Acid Phosphatase 96
Activated clotting time 102
Activated partial thromboplastin time 101
Adenocard 54
Adenosine 7-9, 54
Adjuvants 37
Adrenergic Agonists 74
Aerosol face tent 93
Airway classification 13
Airway Innervation 87
Airway Management 87
Albumin 96
Albumisol 98
Alfentanil 48, 139
Alkaline Phosphatase 96
Allergic Drug Reactions 156
Alprostadil 68
ALT 96
Alveolar uptake 35
Alveolar ventilation 35, 84
American Society of Anesthesiology physical status class 13
Amicar 54, 118
Amidate 61
Aminocaproic Acid 54
Aminophylline 55, 156, 159
Amiodarone 55
Ammonia 96
Amoxicillin 15
Ampicillin 15, 69
Amrinone 55
Amylase 96
Anaphylactoid reactions 156
Anaphylaxis 156
Anesthesia Machine 28, 31
Anesthesia ventilators 28
Anion Gap 86
Anticholinergics 44
Antilirium 67
Anzemet 59
Aorta 122
Apnea of prematurity 112
Apresoline 62
Aprotinin 55, 118
Aqueous Pitressin 151
Arterial Blood Gases 85
Artery of Adamkiewicz 122
Arthritis 12
Aspirin 140
Assist-control ventilation 92
AST 96
Asthma 19
Asystole 6
Ativan 46
Atracurium 41, 110
Atrioventricular Heart Blocks 75

Atropine 6, 7, 9, 14, 44, 56, 110, 115, 146
Automatic Implantable Cardioverter Defibrillator 118
Axillary block 108
Barbiturates 14
Base excess 86
Benadryl 14, 58, 156
Benzodiazepines 45
Bicarbonate 6, 56, 102
Bicarbonate deficit 86
Bicitra 14, 20, 57, 130
Bilirubin 96
Blood 98
Blood volume 98
Body mass index 23, 73
Brachial plexus block 107
Bradycardia 7
Brain death 151
Breathing system 32
Brethine 68
Bretylium 5, 8, 9, 56, 118
Bretylol 56
Brevibloc 60
Brevital 64
Bullard Laryngoscope 95
Bumetanide 56
Bumex 56
Bupivacaine 39, 40, 108, 109, 128, 129, 139
Burns 144
Butorphanol Tartrate 139
Calan 69
Calcium 57, 96, 97, 110
Calcium Chloride 9
Calcium Gluconate 110
Capnogram 29
Carbon Dioxide 27
Carboxyhemoglobin 30
Cardene 65
Cardiac risk factors 16
Cardiac Surgery 114
Cardiac tamponade 145
Cardiopulmonary Resuscitation 5
Cardiovascular Disease 16
Cardiovascular Physiology 72
Cardioversion 8
Cardizem 58
Carotid artery surgery 121
Carotid endarterectomy 121
Cefazolin 69
Cefotetan 69
Central Venous Pressure 77
Cerebral blood flow 133
Cerebral metabolism 134
Cerebral protection 135
Cerebrospinal fluid 133
Cesarean section 129
Chest Radiography 81

Chloral Hydrate 14, 110
Chloride 96
Chloroprocaine 39, 40, 129
Chlorpropamide 21
Cholesterol 96
Chronic obstructive pulmonary disease 19
Cimetidine 14, 130
Cis-atracurium 41
Citrate 57
Clindamycin 15, 69
Closing volume 84
Cocaine 40, 87
Codeine 139
Colloid 98
Combined spinal-epidural block 129
Complete Blood Count 96
Continuous positive airway pressure 92
Controlled mechanical ventilation 92
Cordarone 55
Coronary Perfusion Pressure 73
Creatinine Clearance 72
Croup 113
Cryoprecipitate 98
Crystalloid 98
Cushing reflex 134
Cushing triad 137
Cyclaine 87
Cyclophosphamide 25
Cytoxan 25
d-Tubo-curarine 40, 41
Dantrium 57
Dantrolene 57
Darvon 139
DDAVP 57
Dead space 84
Decadron 57, 135
Demerol 115
Desflurane 52
Desmopressin 57, 118
Dexamethasone 57
Dextran 40 58
Diabetes Mellitus 20
Diabinese 21
Diameter index safety system 28
Diamorphine 138
Diaphragmatic hernia 112
Diazepam 14, 46, 110, 114
Dibucaine 40
Diffusion hypoxia 35
Diflunisal 140
Digoxin 58, 110
Dilaudid 139
Diltiazem 58
Diphenhydramine 58, 106, 159
Dobutamine 9, 59, 74, 110
Dobutrex 59
Dolasetron Mesylate 59

Dopamine 7, 9, 59, 74, 110
Dopexamine 59
Down's Syndrome 12
Doxacurium 40, 41
Drager system 31
Droperidol 59, 110, 141, 154
Ductus arteriosus 114
Ductus venosus 114
Dural puncture 106
Duramorph 129, 130
Dyclone 87
Dyclonine 87
Dymelor 21
Dyshemoglobins 30
Ectopy 8
Edrophonium 45
Edrophonium test 150
EKG changes 76
Elective Cardioversion 120
Electrical Safety 27
Electrical shock 27
Electrocardiograms 74
Electrolyte abnormalities on EKG 75
Electrolytes 97
Elimination half-time 36
Emergency Cardiac Care 5
EMLA 14
Endocarditis Prophylaxis 14
Endocrinology 20
Endotracheal Tube 91
Enflurane 52, 53, 130
Ephedrine 60, 74, 107, 110
Epidural 104, 128
Epiglottis 113
Epinephrine 5-7, 10, 60, 74, 110
Epinephrine, Racemic 60
Epsilon Aminocaproic Acid 118
Ergonovine 60
Ergotrate 60
Erythromycin 15, 69
Esmolol 60, 70
Esophageal Tracheal Combitube 94
Etidocaine 39, 40
Etomidate 50, 61
Extracellular fluid 97
Extubation Criteria 91
Factor VIII deficiency 103
Fail-safe valve 28
Fentanyl 14, 48, 110, 128, 129, 138, 139, 154
Ferritin 96
Fetal circulation 114
Fetal heart monitoring 127
Fick equation 73
Flowmeters 28
Fluids 97
Flumazenil 61
Fluoride induced nephrotoxicity 54
Foramen ovale 114
Fractional Excretion of Sodium 72
Fresh frozen plasma 98
Functional residual capacity 84
Furosemide 61, 102, 110, 135, 155
Gallamine 41
Gas Systems 27
Gastroschisis 113
Gentamicin 15, 69
Glasgow Coma Scale 136
Glipizide 21
Glucose 96, 110
Glucotrol 21
Glyburide 21
Glycopyrrolate 14, 44, 110, 115
Halothane 25, 52, 53
Head trauma 136
HELLP Syndrome 131
Hemodynamic Parameters 72
Hemoglobin Dissociation 83
Hemolytic transfusion reaction 102
Hemophilia A 103
Henderson-Hasselbach equation 86
Heparin 61, 116
Hepatitis B 99
Hepatitis C 99
Hexylcaine 87
High frequency jet ventilation 92
High frequency positive pressure ventilation 92
High frequency ventilation 92
Humalog 21
Hydralazine 62, 70
Hydrocortisone 62
Hydromorphone 138, 139
Hypercalcemia 75
Hypercarbia 85
Hyperkalemia 75
Hypertension 17
Hyperthyroidism 22
Hypertrophic pyloric stenosis 113
Hypocalcemia 75
Hypokalemia 75
Hypothermia 135
Hypothyroidism 23
Ibuprofen 140
Inapsine 141
Indigo Carmine 62
Indigotindisulfonate Sodium 62
Indomethacin 140
Induction Agents 49
Inhaled Anesthetics 51
Inocor 55
Insensible losses 97
Inspiratory force 44
Inspiratory pressure support ventilation 92
Insulin 20, 21, 62, 155
Intermittent mandatory ventilation 92
Intermittent positive-pressure ventilation 92
International normalized ratio 101
Interscalene block 107
Intraaortic balloon pump 81
Intracellular fluid 97
Intracranial pressure 134
Intraocular gas expansion 146
Intraocular pressure 146
Intrathecal block 128
Intropin 59
Intubation 89
Ion trapping 37
Iron 96
Ischemic heart disease 16
Isoflurane 52, 53
Isoproterenol 7, 62, 74, 110
Isuprel 62
Ketamine 14, 50, 62, 110, 130
Ketorolac 63, 140, 149, 154
Labetalol 63, 70, 71, 152
Labor and delivery 127
Laboratory Values 96
Laryngeal Mask Airway 93
Laryngoscope Blade Size 111
Laryngoscope Blade Sizes 91
Laryngospasm 153
Laryngotracheobronchitis 113
Lasix 61
Latex Allergy 157
LDH 96
Lente, NPH 21
Levophed 66
Lidocaine 5, 8-10, 39, 40, 63, 87, 110, 128, 129
Line isolation monitor 27
Liver Disease 25
Local Anesthetics 36
Lopressor 65
Lorazepam 14, 46, 114
Lung Transplantation 125
Machine Check 31
Macintosh blade 89
Macroshock 27
Magnesium 63, 96
Magnesium Sulfate 5, 128, 131
Maintenance Drips 8
Maintenance fluid requirements 97
Malignant Hyperthermia 154
Mannitol 64, 102, 123, 135, 155
Massive transfusion 99
Mechanical Ventilation 92
Meperidine 14, 48, 110, 138, 148, 154
Mepivacaine 39, 40
Metabolic Acidosis 86
Methadone 138

Methemoglobin 30
Methergine 64
Methohexital 14, 64, 110, 148
Methoxyflurane 52, 54
Methyldopa 70, 74
Methylene Blue 64
Methylergonovine 64
Methylprednisolone 65, 137
Metoclopramide 14, 106, 130, 141, 154
Metocurine 40, 41
Metoprolol 65
Metronidazole 69
Micronase 21
Microshock 28
Midazolam 14, 46, 143
Miller blade 89
Milrinone 65
Minimum alveolar concentration 34
Minimum concentration 37
Minute ventilation 84
Mivacurium 41
Mixed Venous Oxygen Saturation 81
Morphine 14, 48, 110, 115, 138, 139, 154
MS Contin 139
Mu receptor 47
Myasthenia Gravis 149
Myasthenic Syndrome 149
Myocardial Ischemia 76
Nalbuphine 106, 139
Naloxone 49, 65, 106, 110
Naproxen 140
Narcan 10, 65
Nasal cannula 93
Nasal intubation 87
Nasotracheal intubation 90
Nasotracheal nerve blocks 87
Nausea 153
Necrotizing enterocolitis 113
Neo-Synephrine 67
Neostigmine 45, 110
Nerve blocks 87
Neuroanesthesia 133
Neuromuscular Blocking Agents 42
Neuromuscular Function Tests 43
Neurotoxicity 38
Newborn Resuscitation 9
Nicardipine 65
Nifedipine 66
Nitrogen 27
Nitroglycerin 66, 70, 117
Nitroprusside 66, 70, 110
Nitrous Oxide 27, 52
Nonobstetric surgery during pregnancy 132
Nonrebreathing mask 93
Norepinephrine 66, 74, 110, 156
Normodyne 63
Nubain 139

Numorphan 139
Obesity 12, 23
Obesity-hypoventilation syndrome 24
Obstetrical Anesthesia 127
Octreotide 66
Oculocardiac reflex 146
Ohmeda system 31
Omphalocele 113
Ondansetron 67
One-lung anesthesia 124
Opioid Antagonist 49
Opioids 47
Organ Harvest 150
Orinase 21
Orotracheal intubation 89
Orotracheal nerve blocks 88
Osmitrol 64
Osmolality 96, 97
Osserman classification 149
Outlet check value 28
Oxycodone HCL 139
Oxygen 27, 93
Oxygen consumption 84
Oxygenation 84
Oxymorphone 138, 139
Oxytocin 67, 127, 130
Pacemakers 76
Packed red blood cells 98
Pain Management 138
Pancuronium 40, 41
Paraplegia 122
Parkland formula 144
Partial pressure 34
Partial rebreathing mask 93
Partial thromboplastin time 101
Patient Controlled Analgesia 138
Patient Monitors 29
Pediatric Airway Management 111
Pediatric Anesthesia 110
Pediatric Endotracheal Tube Sizes 111
Pediatric Vital Signs 111
Pentazocine 138
Pentobarbital 14, 110, 115
Pentothal 49
Penumbra effect 30
Peripartum hemorrhage 132
PGE1 117
Pharmacology 34
Phenergan 14, 68
Phentolamine 70
Phenylephrine 67, 74, 107
Pheochromocytoma 21
Phosphorus 96
Physostigmine 67, 153
Pickwickian syndrome 24
Pin index safety system 28
Pipecuronium 40, 41

Pitocin 67, 127
Pitressin 69
pKa 37
Placenta previa 132
Platelets 98
Pneumonectomy 124
Positive end-expiratory pressure 92
Postanesthesia Care Unit 152
Postdural puncture headache 106
Predicted vital capacity 83
Pregnancy induced hypertension 130
Prematurity 112
Premedications 14
Preoperative Evaluation 11
Preoperative fasting 13
Preoperative interview 11
Pressure regulator 28
Pressure-controlled inverse ratio ventilation 92
Pressure-controlled Ventilation 92
Prilocaine 39, 40
Primacor 65
Procainamide 5, 8, 67
Procaine 39, 40
Procardia 66
Prochlorperazine 154
Promethazine 68, 154
Pronestyl 67
Propofol 51, 68, 93
Propoxyphene HCL 139
Prostaglandin E1 68
Protamine Sulfate 68
Protein 96
Prothrombin time 101
Pulmonary Artery Catheterization 79
Pulmonary Disease 19
Pulmonary function tests 12, 83
Pulse oximetry 30
Pulseless Electrical Activity 6
Pyridostigmine 45, 150
Racemic Epinephrine 153
Ranitidine 14
Rapid Sequence Induction 90
Regional Anesthesia 107
Reglan 141
Remifentanil 48
Respiratory Physiology 83, 84
Retained placenta 132
Retrobulbar block 146, 147
Rheomacrodex 58
Ritodrine 68, 128
Rocuronium 41
Romazicon 61
Safety valves 28
Sandostatin 66
Scavenging system 32
Scleroderma 12
Scopolamine 14, 44, 114
Secobarbital 14

Second gas effect 35
Second stage oxygen pressure regulator 28
Semilente 21
Sevoflurane 52
SGOT 96
SGPT 96
Shivering 153
Sickle Cell Anemia 102
Sodium 96
Sodium Bicarbonate 10, 37, 56, 102, 110, 156
Sodium Thiopental 49
Solu-Medrol 65
SoluCortef 62
Sonoclot 101
Sphenopalatine ganglion 87
Spinal Anesthesia 104
Spinal cord injury 137
Stadol 139
STP 110
Succinylcholine 40-42, 110
Sufenta 48
Sufentanil 14, 128, 129, 138, 139
Supraclavicular block 107
Synchronized intermittent mandatory ventilation 92
Tachycardia 7
Terbutaline 68, 128
Tetanic stimulation 43, 44
Tetracaine 39, 40, 87, 108
Thoracic Surgery 124
Thromboelastrogram 101
Tidal volume 43, 84
Tobramycin 70
Tocolytics 128
Tolazamide 21
Tolbutamide 21
Tolinase 21
Total body bicarbonate deficit 86
Total body water 97
Tracheal intubation 88, 91
Tracheoesophageal fistula 113
Train-of-four 44
Trandate 63
Tranexamic Acid 118
Transfusion reaction 99
Transtracheal Ventilation 91
Trasylol 55
Trauma 142
Triglycerides 96
Trimethaphan 70
Twitch height 43
Tylenol 110
Ultiva 48
Ultralente 21
Uric Acid 96
Urolene Blue 64
Uterine atony 132
Uterine inversion 132
Uterine rupture 132
Valium 10, 46

Valvular Heart Disease 115
Vancomycin 15, 70
Vaponefrin 60
Vaporizers 28
Variable bypass 28
Vasa previa 132
Vascular Surgery 121
Vasopressin 69
Vecuronium 41, 110
Venous Air Embolism 156
Venous oximetry 81
Ventilation 84
Ventilator Settings 93
Ventricular Ectopy 8
Ventricular Fibrillation 5
Ventricular Tachycardia 5
Venturi mask 93
Verapamil 7, 69, 110
Versed 46, 110
Vinblastine 25
Vincristine 25
Vistaril 14
Vital capacity 43, 84
Volume of distribution 36
Vomiting 153
Whole Blood 98
Yutopar 68
Zofran 67

Titles from Current Clinical Strategies Publishing

In Bookstores Worldwide

Medicine, 1998 Edition
Pediatrics 5 Minute Review, 1998-99 Edition
Anesthesiology, 1999-2000 Edition
Handbook of Psychiatric Drugs, 1998-99 Edition
Gynecology and Obstetrics, 1999-2000 Edition
Manual of HIV/AIDS Therapy, 1997 Edition
Family Medicine, 1997 Edition
Practice Parameters in Medicine and Primary Care, 1999-2000 Edition
Surgery, 1999-2000 Edition
Pediatric Drug Reference, 1996 Edition
Critical Care Medicine, 1997 Edition
Outpatient Medicine, 1997 Edition
History and Physical Examination in Medicine, Second Edition
Psychiatry, 1999-2000 Edition
Pediatrics, 1997 Edition
Physicians' Drug Resource, 1997 Edition

Windows/Macintosh CD-ROM and Softcover Book

Internet Journals from Current Clinical Strategies Publishing

Journal of Primary Care Medicine
Journal of Medicine
Journal of Pediatric Medicine
Journal of Surgery
Journal of Family Medicine
Journal of Emergency Medicine and Acute Primary Care
Journal of Psychiatry
Journal of AIDS/HIV

www.ccspublishing.com